Handbook of Health Evangelism

Handbook of Health Evangelism

Elvin Adams, MD, MPH

iUniverse, Inc.
New York Lincoln Shanghai

Handbook of Health Evangelism

iUniverse, Inc.

For information address:
iUniverse, Inc.
2021 Pine Lake Road, Suite 100
Lincoln, NE 68512
www.iuniverse.com

All quotations from Ellen White's *Spirit of Prophecy* books were previously published by the Review and Herald Publishing Association.

ISBN: 0-595-31243-8

Printed in the United States of America

Contents

Foreword

Earnest Christians recognize and value the close relationship that exists between the physical, mental, and spiritual nature of humans. Such believers have frequently sought to share these insights with their neighbors and friends so they too can experience vibrant physical health, dynamic mental and social well-being, and fulfilling spiritual growth and happiness. In so doing, they have expanded the traditional meaning of evangelism to include the whole person.

In the past few decades the topic of Health Evangelism has captured the imagination and attention of many who desire to share their Christian faith in ways that are more effective than traditional evangelistic methods. These efforts have been many and varied. Some evangelists have invited health professionals to give short "health nuggets" prior to the main presentation, often emphasizing the health appeal in the advertising. Others have sought to prepare the ground by general or specific sequences of health programming in the community prior to evangelistic outreach. Still others have conducted excellent health education programs in churches and community halls without any overt evangelistic connection to create a positive public relations impact. And of course, some programs have been conducted so unscientifically or so dogmatically that they turn off any interest the participants might have in further association with church activities!

Today traditional evangelism faces significant challenges, especially in the more secular and affluent parts of the globe. Methods that used to attract hundreds, even thousands of attendees, with large numbers baptized are only marginally successful in these endeavors. Many are asking what the solution could be.

While there has been much experimentation and high expectations generated for Health Evangelism, most pastors and evangelists dismiss it as largely ineffective in swelling the numbers of converts. Yes, there have been successful examples of this kind of work, but they are unfortunately few and far between.

Those successful efforts that are operated on sound principles, built on a careful understanding of the whole process of evangelism, a correct understanding of the role Health Evangelism plays, mixed with a large dose of genuine love for others.

As this book so eloquently points out, Health Evangelism will never reach its true potential until we stop conducting independent events, no matter how well they are done—and take to heart the fact that evangelism is a process that involves many significant events and stages in the life of the potential convert. This process can take place in a matter of a few months, but more often requires years to reach full fruition.

I have had the privilege of being personally acquainted with Dr. Adams for more than 30 years. His professional training, life experiences and passion for Health Evangelism uniquely qualify him to author this book. I was a graduate student at Loma Linda University when I first heard him speak on this topic, and my heart was thrilled. Since that time we have both learned much! While the opportunities to collaborate together in Health Evangelism activities have been disappointingly few, I cherish equally his thoughtful advice and warm Christian friendship. When I have ignored his suggestions I usually have come to regret it!

Having been personally involved in Health Evangelism in North America and internationally for more than 25 years, I am thrilled to see this book published. It is a long time overdue. Dr. Adams powerfully captures the essence of Health Evangelism, aptly describing in proper perspective the length and breadth of such activities, and provides very practical advice on how to organize and conduct effective programs in your church and community. You will refer to it over and over.

I commend this book to anyone interested in becoming a more effective soul-winner. By following the principles found within these pages you will see your soul-winning efforts multiply many fold. There is no better reward!

Fred Hardinge, DrPH, RD
It Is Written Television International
Director, Bibleinfo.com

(Former Health Ministries Director for Potomac Conference, Far Eastern Division, Upper Columbia Conference.)

1

What is Health Evangelism?

Health evangelism is a ministry that changes people. Health evangelism improves health, prevents disease and lengthens life. Health evangelism results in a knowledge of and a deeper experience with God. Health evangelism results in baptisms and church growth. Health evangelism is the right arm of the gospel.

Unfortunately, health evangelism is misunderstood and poorly practiced by the Seventh-day Adventist church. From time to time, in various places a few health professionals, a few pastors and a few church members have developed and conducted health evangelism programs. Some health evangelism activities enjoyed a few months or years of success but most of these activities were local in their effect and never achieved national or international success. The 5-Day Plan to Stop Smoking is an exception. It achieved international status. Most of these programs and efforts have faded and have died out.

For more than 30 years I have talked up health evangelism. I have conducted a wide variety of health evangelism programs in hospitals, churches, private homes, and public places. I have worked in the United States and promoted health evangelism in nearly a dozen countries. I have always felt called by God to do this.

Over the years I have worked for local churches, state conferences and the Health Ministries Department of the General Conference. I have worked for self-supporting institutions and more than one large hospital. I have been on the faculty of schools of public health and am on the faculty of a local medical school at present. I am currently working in the Public Health Department of a large city.

It is my assessment that health evangelism, to this point, has largely been a failure for the Seventh-day Adventist church. It wasn't supposed to be this way. I still think health evangelism will eventually be done right. I have a vision of how health evangelism should be done.

That is why I am writing this book. I have prayed about health evangelism. I have studied health evangelism in scripture and the writings of Ellen White. I have organized and practiced health evangelism in many different ways.

This book summarizes what I have learned that works and what doesn't work for me. If you are a pastor, layperson or health professional, interested in the health message of the Seventh-day Adventist church and how to share this with others, this book is for you. I hope and pray that you will put these principles to work. God will bless you.

In my practice of health evangelism I have been inspired most by the healing ministry of our Lord and Savior Jesus Christ who spent more time healing than in preaching. I have been inspired by the picture of health evangelism outlined in Isaiah 58 and certain key passages in the Spirit of Prophecy.

The quotation that most intrigues me is: " I wish to tell you that soon there will be no work done in ministerial lines but medical missionary work…" Counsels on Health 533. This brief passage tells me that medical missionary work will eclipse everything that ministers are now doing in the church.

This could mean that the obvious spiritual part of the church's work will become so prohibited that at some point in time a more subtle secondary way of doing pastoral work in the guise of health evangelism will be the only course open for evangelization. A sort of "second-best but it will have to do" type of development.

I believe the church will eventually find that medical missionary work is a *superior* form of evangelism not just a "second best" effort. Evangelistic efforts characterized by traditional doctrinal presentations appear to work well in some parts of the world but traditional evangelistic efforts are much less effective in the United States, western Europe, Australia and Japan.

If it is true that soon there will be no work done in ministerial lines but medical missionary work shouldn't we be exploring ways of maximizing the effectiveness of health evangelism now? We should be experimenting with medical missionary work. We should work at it until health evangelism is a tool that we find surpasses the effectiveness of traditional evangelistic approaches.

When the superior effectiveness of health evangelism is demonstrated, we will switch over to the better way of doing things. I hope this happens soon so the work can be done and we can go home to Heaven.

Here is a second quotation from the Spirit of Prophecy that has challenged me.

> "Again and again I have been instructed that the medical missionary work is to bear the same relation to the work of the third angel's message that the arm and hand bear to the body. Under the direction of the divine Head they are to work unitedly in preparing the way for the coming of Christ. The right arm of the body of truth is to be constantly active, constantly at work, and God will

strengthen it. But it is not to be made the body. At the same time the body is not to say to the arm: "I have no need of thee." The body has need of the arm in order to do active, aggressive work. Both have their appointed work, and each will suffer great loss if worked independently of the other." Testimonies for the Church Volume Six, 288.

This vision of health evangelism just hasn't happened. Some among us see a fulfillment of this in our current Adventist Health System. The plain truth is that, in the United States, the hospitals operated by the Seventh-day Adventist church are not efficient evangelistic tools for the church. Our hospitals are deeply in debt and many are struggling, along with the rest of the hospitals in the nation, to stay afloat financially. Additionally, there is no meaningful connection between hospitals and church evangelistic activities.

Oh yes, we have church officials sitting of the boards of hospitals. This doesn't count for much. This doesn't make hospitals particularly Christian or Adventist. Hospital patients aren't flocking in great numbers to evangelistic efforts. Hospitals are great healing institutions and evangelistic efforts set forth the doctrines of the church but these separate efforts to make man whole are on different tracks and there is no viable connection between the two.

One prominent hospital administrator told me. "When the finances get tight, something has to go and it is going to be health education and preventive medicine." Adventist hospitals haven't been the soul winning right arm they were envisioned to be. Our hospitals are staffed largely with well-trained non-Adventist physicians and nurses and provide a level of health care that is about average for what is available at other secular hospitals in the community. There will be more to say about the Adventist hospitals later in this book.

It is my contention today, that the right arm of the message has been severed from the body and is functioning independently. Both the body and the arm have suffered great loss by having worked independently of each other and I see greater loss in the future.

The quote from Spirit of Prophecy which most clearly points out where health evangelism should be done and who should be doing it is:

"We have come to a time when *every member* of the church should take hold of medical missionary work. The world is a lazar house filled with victims of both physical and spiritual disease. Everywhere people are perishing for lack of a knowledge of the truths that have been committed to us. *The members of the church* are in need of an awakening, that they may realize their responsibility to impart these truths." Welfare Ministry, p. 138

Here the root of our current problem is outlined. We haven't been doing health evangelism in the right place. The institution in which health evangelism is to occur is the *local church*. The home of health evangelism is not to be hospitals, schools, public auditoriums, outpost centers, or better living centers but the local church.

This quotation also indicates who is to do health evangelism. *Every member* of the church should take hold of medical missionary work. There is a role for pastors, doctors, dentists, nurses, therapists, counselors and others but every church member needs to be involved with health evangelism.

Part of the problem is that health professionals have tried to organize and conduct health evangelism programs independent of the church and church members. Most of the time this limits church member support to contributing some money, sitting in the pew or praying for the program's success. Health evangelism conducted in this way fails to create an interface between the church member and the pubic. This is a serious mistake.

As a church we have tried to become more popular. By relaxing standards and adopting many of the ways of the world, we hope to make the Seventh-day Adventist Church more palatable to our friends in the community. There is a better way to correct misconceptions and attract people in the community. Our neighbors will value our church more if we learn to do health evangelism in the right way. Health evangelism removes prejudice that exists against the church.

> "Much of the prejudice that prevents the truth of the third angel's message from reaching the hearts of the people might be removed if more attention were given to health reform. When people become interested in this subject, the way is often prepared for the entrance of other truths. If they see that we are intelligent with regard to health, they will be more ready to believe that we are sound in Bible doctrines." Counsels on Health, p. 452

Has health evangelism ever been done right? I think the closest example I can find is the Weigh Down program developed by Ms. Shamblin. It is a weight loss program that has swept the nation. It is spiritually based. At its peak there were more than 10,000 chapters in the United States. It is conducted largely in churches by church members. It is an example of what God can do when His model is followed.

I hope we as a people will learn to do health evangelism in the right way. Let's follow the counsel that has been given us. Let us design and conduct programs that will utilize church members, be conducted in the local church and be aggressively evangelistic.

As you read these pages I hope God will impress your mind with the importance of health evangelism. I hope you will be inspired to implement health evangelism in your local church and that the third angel's message will be completed in your community due to your efforts and the efforts of your fellow church members.

2

The Soul Winning Connection

Where Are the Baptisms?

Over the years of conducting health evangelism programs I have repeatedly been asked, "Where are the baptisms?" This is a fair question. Pastors and church administrators are interested in numbers that indicate church growth. Church membership is rapidly expanding around the world. A person is counted as an authentic member once baptism has taken place. There is a heavy emphasis on baptisms. What is the relationship between health evangelism and baptisms? Should you expect baptisms from health evangelism programs? Read on.

In the past, health education programs weren't particularly evangelistic. Many health education programs were conducted in an entirely secular manner in a secular setting. It would not be expected that these would be evangelistic in any way or result in baptisms. These more secular programs were rightly accused of making "healthy sinners."

Other health education programs were integrated in some way with traditional evangelistic efforts. In some cases a Five-day Plan to Stop Smoking was held just before an evangelistic crusade in the hopes that the reformed smokers would stay for the doctrinal presentations once they stopped smoking. This never worked very well.

At other times a health segment was included in an evangelistic crusade. A "health nugget" would come before the real meat of the program. This format sometimes increased the crowds, and reformed health habits but there was only a marginal increase in baptisms.

Over time most evangelists, not seeing any particular baptismal benefit from health education, abandoned the combination of the health message with evangelistic efforts. With the gradual secularization of the church membership at many levels, the whole health message of the church has been pretty much abandoned by pastors and church administrators.

The problem is not with health evangelism as much as it is with traditional evangelism. What worked well in the United States 75 years ago, is no longer effective in drawing crowds into the church. Large public evangelistic efforts are effective in developing countries and should continue to be conducted in those settings. In developed countries where traditional evangelistic crusades have been shown to be ineffective, new strategies need to be considered. I believe it is time to take a fresh look at health evangelism.

Friendship Evangelism

Health evangelism programs, rightly conducted, will lead to baptisms and will elevate the reputation of a church in the community. Health evangelism programs, organized along the lines suggested in this book will make many friends in the community and go a long ways toward preparing people for baptism and full church membership.

A survey of recent converts to the church in North America identified the various reasons a person joined a church. This is the data.

1.	Friends	79%
2.	Pastor	6%
3.	Sabbath School	5%
4.	Programs	3%
5.	Special need	2%
6.	Visitation	1%
7.	Crusade	1%

The most important influence in a person joining a church is the presence of friends in the congregation. Health evangelism programs, when conducted in the way recommended in this book, creates friends. Health evangelism programs should be designed to create an interface between church members and the community.

Soul saving friendships occur in small groups that meet each session of the program. Lasting friendships with men and women from the community have been formed in every group I have organized. From these friendships new church members are acquired.

Traditional evangelistic efforts are usually conducted by a charismatic preacher who carries the burden of presenting truth pretty much by himself or herself. Usually, there are no small groups and no meaningful interface between church members and the public who come to these large meetings. Almost every year now, there are evangelistic efforts that are spread around the world by satellite down links. Thousands of churches can receive the evangelistic message simultaneously. This has resulted in tens of thousands of baptism.

In traditional evangelistic efforts, if church members are involved from a local congregation, they are usually relegated to the role of helping to swell the audience, perhaps usher or take up the offering. There is no specific activity in traditional evangelistic meetings designed for individuals from the public to create friendships with church members from the local congregation. This is one of the reasons why so many new members leave the church shortly after the meetings are past. They simply don't have any friends in the church. They get baptized into a church of strangers.

New church members are more likely to stay if they have at least one good friend in the church. Health evangelism programs create one-on-one relationships and sustain them as solid friendships are formed. Baptisms that result from health evangelism programs where friendships are made, are much more likely to stay in the church than baptisms resulting from traditional evangelistic activities.

Health evangelism programs will prepare community people to be exposed to more traditional evangelistic meetings at some subsequent time. Health evangelism and traditional evangelistic meetings should not be piggy backed one on the other but each should be conducted often enough that those who are ready for indoctrination can avail themselves of a traditional evangelistic crusade.

What I am calling for is health evangelism on one continuing track and traditional evangelistic efforts at regular intervals on another track. The purpose of each track is clear. The health evangelism track is health oriented but creates firm friendships with church members and introduces a person to God as the agent of behavior change in the daily life. The traditional evangelistic crusade track is for the purpose of broadening the religious understanding experience of an individual along doctrinal lines. This prepares a person for membership in the church. More about these parallel tracks in a later chapter.

Baptism: Event or Process

Baptism is an event that can be easily quantified. Before baptism, you are not a member of the church. After baptism you are a member in full and regular standing. Baptisms are counted and the quality of a pastor's ministry is often equated with the number of baptisms that are performed during the past year. This is tragic because it ignores the long process that leads up to baptism and also ignores the process of discipling that should follow baptism.

Becoming a Christian is not an event but a lengthy process. Baptism is a point along a continuum. We put too much emphasis on baptism and tend to ignore the process. There are many points along the process to baptism that can be measured. Health evangelism programs lead people through many of these points and move an audience well along the process toward baptism.

Those who conduct health evangelism programs should measure all of these intermediate steps that lead to baptism. When this is done, the value of health evangelism will be seen by pastors and church administrators and a renewed interest in health evangelism will result. What are these intermediate steps?

Step 1 Leading to Baptism: Interest in something you do in your church. What does your church do? Sabbath services are probably the most notable thing your church does. Frankly, services in your church won't be of much interest to anyone who goes to their own church on a regular basis. Go to church here or go church there, who cares as long as you go.

Health evangelism will make your church much more attractive because few churches do anything for the health of the community. If your church regularly helped people stop smoking, that would make your church more attractive to the smokers in your community. If your church regularly helped obese people lose weight, that would make your church more attractive to the obese people in your community. If your church sponsored an Alcoholics Anonymous program on a regular basis that would make your church attractive to the alcoholics in your community.

The more health evangelism activities you conduct, in your church on a regular basis, the more interest the community will have in your church. This would simply be a social gospel if your help was solely physical or mental in nature. If your community activities point to God as the agent of lasting behavior change in the human life, then they become health evangelism activities.

The very first step in a person becoming a member of your church is an interest in something you do in your church. So, start doing something. Do it often, do it well and do it regularly and the community will flock to your church. This step in the process of becoming a church member is difficult to measure but can be determined by surveys of community knowledge and attitudes about your church.

Step 2 Leading to Baptism: Come to your church. This is another obvious step in becoming a church member. Health evangelism programs help people take this step if they are conducted in the local church. When a person comes to a health evangelism program in your church they must get directions, drive to your church, find a parking spot, find the right entrance, come through the door, and say "hello."

Of course, this is what every member does every time they come to church. It is much less threatening for a person in the community, whether they are a member of another church or never go to church, to come to your church for a health evangelism program than to come to regular religious services on the weekend.

If you provide specific help for a specific health problem at your church, the community will come. At some time in the future, when they have made friends with the church members who are helping you conduct the health evangelism program, they will find it much easier to come to your church for religious services because they know how to get to your church, they know where to park, which door to come through, they will recognize people and will even know where the restrooms are.

This step toward baptism is as easy to measure as baptisms. Keeping statistics on the number of non-church member visits to your church will be a measure of the effectiveness of your health evangelism program. These numbers will help pastors and church administrators see the value of your health evangelism program.

I advise you to measure every visit by every non-church member every time they step through your door. If 20 non-church members attend a 5-Day Plan to Stop smoking for 5 nights that equals 100 non-church member visits to your church.

Step 3 Leading to Baptism: Become friends with church members. I will have much more to say about this later, but for now, let me say that health evangelism programs can be conducted in the same impersonal way that many evangelistic crusades are. This has been a design flaw in many health evangelism programs as well. Most health education programs have been designed to provide accurate health and medical information but have been poor at providing personal contact with church members. I believe that health evangelism programs should be designed to maximize the interface with church members. This is the one factor that will change them from being primarily informational to being interactive and evangelistic.

Each church member who helps with your health evangelism program should be assigned to 3-4 community participants. Sufficient time should be created in the health Evangelism program for church members to interact with the individuals from the community. Give church members real but simple work to do. Let them review the high points of the night's lecture. Let them ask individuals what they personally have decided to do in their own lives as a result of the lecture.

Give the church members time to get some feedback from the participants in small groups. Let them listen to their struggles and hardships. Teach them to have a sympathetic ear. Teach them to be nonjudgmental. Teach them to be friends. This is not hard for church members to learn or to do. This type of friendship activity is not at all like giving formal Bible studies. Give church members a list of questions to ask and teach them to listen and be sympathetic. This is how friendships are formed.

This is a step toward baptism that can be measured. Count each church member contact with a non-church member in a small group as a friendship interaction. This is another step toward baptism that results from health evangelism programs.

Step 4 Leading to Baptism: Develop or strengthen a relationship with God. This is probably the most important step in any health evangelism program. If you become a church member without taking this step you are a Christian only in name. We expect that church membership is equated with a personal relationship with God. Where and when does this relationship with God occur? Baptism is the public step that indicates that an individual has made a full commitment to God but baptism doesn't make it happen.

Health evangelism programs are an ideal setting for a person to get to know God. People come to health evangelism programs because they have a behavioral problem that needs to be changed. In the program you provide information that confirms that your audience needs to change. You provide individual counseling and friendship through your church members but the audience needs more.

In every health evangelism program there should be simple, specific information on how God helps people change behavior. This evangelistic approach should be very specific and narrowly focused on the behavioral problem the participant is trying to overcome. Many will find that God is an ever present help in time of need in a health evangelism program if you design it that way.

Information about God, with an opportunity to apply His help to a specific problem, puts evangelism into health education and creates a health evangelism program. If a person doesn't find God's help with a problem when they attend your health evangelism program, why should they ever decide to become a member of your church? On the other hand, If a person does find that God helps them in tangible ways in a health evangelism program they will be much more inclined to join your church once they have been introduced to the distinctive doctrines at some subsequent evangelistic meeting.

This step toward baptism can be measured but is a bit more difficult. In your exit questionnaire, following a health evangelism program, and in each of the follow-up visits with participants you can ask what their relationship with God is with respect to the problem they were trying to overcome. Many will confess that they have a new or deeper relationship with God as a result of your health evangelism program. They will concede that they never would have been successful in changing their behavior unless they had received God's help.

This is one more step in the process leading to baptism. We shouldn't baptize anyone who doesn't have an experimental knowledge of God. Too often we baptize people who intellectually give assent to a body of doctrines but who have no real experience of God's power in their lives.

Step 5 Leading to Baptism: Changing certain behaviors. This is not as much a step leading to baptism as it used to be. There is much less emphasis on healthful living than there used to be. Baptismal candidates aren't held accountable for health behaviors as much as they were in the past. People don't have to give up flesh foods, coffee, tea or caffeine containing beverages. We still discourage smoking but moderate alcohol use is wide spread in the church today. Just at a time when we know so much about healthful living it seems to be less important in the lives of church members and is a diminishing part of our evangelistic thrust.

Obviously, health evangelism programs are about changing the way you live. Many health destroying habits and addictions can be changed in a health evangelism program. A new healthier lifestyle is another step toward baptism and it is quite easy to measure.

Step 6 Leading to Baptism: Accept Distinctive Doctrines. This is the last step in the process leading to baptism. To be a church member in regular standing it is necessary to accept the distinctive doctrines of the church. This is *not* a function of health evangelism with the exception of those distinctive health doctrines having to do with healthful living. This is the domain of traditional evangelism in its various forms.

Step 7 Leading to Church Membership: Baptism. At last, a person joins the church by baptism. We all rejoice! This is the main goal of the church. The church is to proclaim the gospel of Jesus Christ and to baptize those who believe on His name.

Is it fair to ask those who conduct health evangelism programs, "Where are the baptisms?" Not really. The question reveals an ignorance of the processes that leads to baptism. Such a question reveals a lack of appreciation for the many ways in which health evangelism prepares people for baptism. Out of the seven steps leading to baptism I have outlined above, health evangelism leads people through the first five. That should be good enough. That is all that health evangelism rightly designed and conducted will do.

Health evangelism is only the right hand of the gospel not the whole gospel. Health evangelism opens doors, makes friends, gives them an experimental relationship with God but it does not and should not result directly in baptisms.

Health evangelism programs should be understood as "problem specific" evangelism. It is getting saved over just one behavioral problem, not all of life's problems. The saved all started their journey to God at some point. Health evangelism can be the starting point for many. A rudimentary experience with God, developed in overcoming a specific health problem, can lead to a fuller experience in all areas of life.

Your church should hold health evangelism programs that are designed and conducted in the way that will guide people in the steps leading to baptism. Do not say that health evangelism programs are not evangelistic. They can be and they are. It is a focused evangelism that helps people deal with specific addictions and habits.

I had one lady who had successfully quit smoking with God's help. After several weeks she correctly observed, "This is a model of behavior change that I can now apply to other areas in my life." That would be sanctification in more traditional theological terms. She had learned that God had helped her with one problem and she was now ready to expand her experience with God and overcome in other areas as well.

Disinterested Service

Over the years, I have met resistance from pastors, laymen and health professionals about putting even problem specific evangelism into the health program. The objection raised is that we are supposed to be providing "disinterested service." The thought being that we are to provide for the specific physical or psychological needs of individuals who come to health programs without regard to our specific interest in them joining our church. Why bother someone about spiritual matters when all they wanted to do is stop smoking? The following quotes from Spirit of Prophecy are used to support the position of those who want to leave spiritual issues out of health education programs. These passages require some comment.

> "In your care of the sick, act tenderly, kindly, faithfully, that you may have a converting influence upon them. You have need of the grace of Christ in order to properly represent the service of Christ. And as you present the grace of truth in true *disinterested service*, angels will be present to sustain you. The Comforter will be with you to fulfill the promise of the Saviour, "Lo, I am with you alway, even unto the end of the world." Medical Ministry, p. 196

Disinterested service doesn't mean that we act without regard to the spiritual needs of people. Disinterested service means we don't perform acts of charity for selfish purposes, personal gain or recognition. Some would say that inserting an evangelistic component in a health education program represents a selfish purpose but this is not the case.

The passage above specifically mentions that disinterested service may result in a "converting influence," we are to represent the "grace of truth." Presenting spiritual matters is not a selfish matter. It is a matter of eternal importance and should be free of any personal wishes for recognition and not mixed with desire for enrichment or personal gain.

> "The Lord sees and understands, and He will use you, despite your weakness, if you offer your talent as a consecrated gift to His service; for in active, *disinterested service* the weak become strong and enjoy His precious commendation. The joy of the Lord is an element of strength. If you are faithful, the peace that passeth all understanding will be your reward in this life, and in the future life you will enter into the joy of your Lord. Christian Service, 101.

In this quotation we see that even though we may be weak, as we dedicate our skills to His service, free from selfish purposes for things like personal gain or recognition, the Lord strengthens us to do His service.

In the following quotation, disinterested service is seen to include such things as praying with people, reading to them from the Bible, and speaking with them of the Saviour. This is specifically with regard to the control of appetite. So, there is no place for excluding God as the agent of behavior change in the name of conducting health programs with "disinterested service."

> "In almost every community there are large numbers who do not listen to the preaching of God's word or attend any religious service. If they are reached by the gospel, it must be carried to their homes. Often the relief of their physical needs is the only avenue by which they can be approached. Missionary nurses who care for the sick and relieve the distress of the poor will find many opportunities to *pray with them*, to *read to them from God's word*, and to *speak of the*

Saviour. They can pray with and for the helpless ones who have not strength of will to control the appetites that passion has degraded. They can bring a ray of hope into the lives of the defeated and disheartened. Their unselfish love, manifested in acts of *disinterested kindness*, will make it easier for the suffering ones to believe in the love of Christ." Messages to Young People, p. 223

Next we see that disinterested service includes denying self to do good for others, devoting all we have to the service of Christ and not laying up treasures for ourselves on earth by avoiding the love of money. Nothing is said about leaving a spiritual message out of our efforts.

"Those who deny self to do others good, and who devote themselves and all they have to Christ's service, will realize the happiness which the selfish man seeks for in vain. Said our Saviour: "Whosoever he be of you that forsaketh not all that he hath, he cannot be My disciple." Charity "seeketh not her own." This is the fruit of that *disinterested* love and benevolence which characterized the life of Christ. The law of God in our hearts will bring our own interests in subordination to high and eternal considerations. We are enjoined by Christ to seek first the kingdom of God and His righteousness. This is our first and highest duty. Our Master expressly warned His servants not to lay up treasures upon the earth; for in so doing their hearts would be upon earthly rather than heavenly things. Here is where many poor souls have made shipwreck of faith. They have gone directly contrary to the express injunction of our Lord, and have allowed the love of money to become the ruling passion of their lives. They are intemperate in their efforts to acquire means. They are as much intoxicated with their insane desire for riches as is the inebriate with his liquor." Testimonies for the Church Volume Three, 397-398.

It is often necessary to meet the temporal necessities of the individuals we help. We may need to provide clothing, food or shelter. But in the process, we should look for the opportunity to speak of virtue and the love of Christ. Disinterested service will not purposely leave out opportunities to speak a word for God.

"Thy neighbor as thyself,"—the question arises, "Who is my neighbor?" The Saviour's reply is found in the parable of the good Samaritan, which teaches us that any human being who needs our sympathy and our kind offices, is our neighbor. The suffering and destitute of all classes are our neighbors; and when their wants are brought to our knowledge it is our duty to relieve them as far as possible. A principle is brought out in this parable that it would be well for the followers of Christ to adopt. First meet the temporal necessities of the needy, and relieve their physical wants and sufferings, and you will then find an open avenue to the heart, where you may plant the good seeds of virtue and religion." Advent Review and Sabbath Herald, 01-18-1887.

The church has been asked to provide services of a humanitarian nature in developing countries. At times contracts with governments prohibit any active proselytizing. The name of Jesus can't be named, prayers can't be offered and spiritual meetings can't be held. It is my opinion that sinking resources into such operations doesn't represent disinterested service.

In circumstances where proclaiming the gospel is specifically prohibited, when we agree to limit our efforts to secular activities, we are no better than any other worldly enterprise that provides physical services. If we feel constrained or are contractually constrained from speaking freely about God when circumstances warrant and opportunity occurs, we should avoid those opportunities and let others carry on that work.

Evangelism is the work of the church in all of its institutional settings. The health work should never be an exception. Health ministry in all forms should be designed to be evangelistic. Evangelistic opportunities should be maximized. Questions need to be asked at every juncture. "Will this element increase or decrease the evangelistic potential of this enterprise?"

Summary

1. Health evangelism creates an interest in something you do in your church.

2. Health evangelism attracts people to come to your church.

3. Health evangelism creates friendships between church members and the public.

4. Health evangelism helps people develop a closer relationship with God.

5. Health evangelism helps people change certain health destroying behaviors.

6. Health evangelism does not introduce, review or cover distinctive doctrines.

7. Health evangelism does not directly result in baptisms but does move people through five of the seven steps leading to baptism.

8. Disinterested service includes talking of God, praying and putting Christianity right in the middle of health evangelism activities.

9. Disinterested service excludes selfish, profit making, self-seeking motivation in doing health evangelism.

3

Types of Programs

This is a review of a few of the various types of health education programs that have been developed by others. There have been a variety of formats and settings for health education. Here are the strengths and weaknesses I recognize in each approach.

Local Church-based Programs

Health evangelism programs have occasionally been conducted in the local church. The next chapter deals with the advantages and desirability of working in the local church. The denomination has more churches than any other type of institution. There are currently 50,000 Seventh-day Adventist Churches. Church buildings are designed to hold group meetings. Church buildings stand empty most of the time. This creates an ideal setting for health evangelism.

Church-based programs have included smoking cessation programs, weight management programs, nutrition courses and cooking schools. The programs don't cater to the sick, offering them a cure, as much as they do to the worried well who have bad habits and behaviors that will destroy health if not corrected.

An example of a church-based program is the Coronary Health Improvement Project (CHIP). This is a program that focuses on reducing coronary heart disease and includes principles that help people reduce their risk of diabetes and obesity. A number of churches across the United States have been successfully conducting CHIP in their communities. This program relies on a series of videos and handout materials produced by Hans Diehl, DHSc. An excellent program manual is available from the Adventist CHIP Association as well as personal instruction and counsel on how to conduct one of these intense (four nights per week) month-long program.

Churches conducting CHIP enter into a contractual arrangement that limits the area where the videos can be used by a church and requires that $25.00 per attendee be returned to CHIP. This program does not have material on how God helps with behavior change. The overt spiritual content is minimal.

Some programs are probably not appropriate for a local church setting. Drug rehabilitation should probably not be done in the local church. Drug addicts often need to be institutionalized to get them off drugs. Drug addicts need frequent monitoring and support services for an extended period of time. The local church might have a prevention or maintenance program but not a drug detoxification program.

The same might be true for alcoholism. The church might sponsor an Alcoholics Anonymous program but leave acute detoxification to hospitals. If your church does sponsor an AA meeting, I believe it should be a nonsmoking meeting where coffee, tea and caffeine drinks are not provided or allowed.

Some churches have sponsored medical clinics for the poor. I currently volunteer at Mission Fort Worth. This is a medical clinic sponsored by a Baptist Church. Indigent members of the community are well served by this clinic. It does require a high level of security to protect supplies of medications. This clinic requires the services of physicians and nurses. There are liability issues that come up with this type of clinic as well. Providing clinical care would only be appropriate for a few churches. The spiritual needs of patients are addressed through staff who pray with those who come for treatment. Clinic patients are also invited to Bible Studies and church services. The Church is right across the street from the clinic.

Hospital-based Health evangelism

Hospitals don't do much in the way of health education or health evangelism. The Lankenau hospital in Philadelphia (An institution with Lutheran roots) has the most developed health education program I have seen. They have a huge health museum and students from surrounding school districts tour the facilities regularly. It is open to the public. While this is an excellent example of health education, it really isn't health evangelism.

Hospitals have conducted smoking cessation programs with some success. The very first 5-Day Plan to Stop Smoking program I ever helped conduct was with Elder A. C. Marple, Chaplin of the Washington Adventist Hospital. This was in the late 60's and smoking cessations clinics in those days were well attended. We had 40-60 participants attending every session in a hospital conference room.

This 5-Day Plan to Stop Smoking at the Washington Adventist Hospital helped the hospital's reputation in the community. Elder Marple made the program slightly evangelistic by referring to help that was available from God but no specifics or "how to" instructions were given.

The disadvantage of the hospital-based program was that there was no connection with the local church. There were no church members to be buddies with those who were trying to quit. Elder Marple wasn't a pastor of a congregation. There was no follow-up. In short, there was no way to connect smokers with a local church for their continued spiritual growth.

Health education programs in hospitals have tended toward rehabilitation services for specific conditions. There is diabetic education concerning home blood sugar testing and details of the diabetic diet. There is cardiac rehabilitation for those who have had a heart attack. This includes dietary recommendations and a graduated exercise program under controlled and monitored conditions. This helps define the limits within which a cardiac patient can work or exercise.

Some hospitals have pulmonary rehabilitation programs for those with emphysema or chronic bronchitis who have stopped smoking but need continued lung treatments and breathing exercises. Smoking education and cessation advice are also provided.

Some hospitals provide grief recovery for spouses and family members after losing a loved one. All of these activities are especially suited for hospitals. The spiritual dimensions of these various health problems are not addressed and the educators are often not members of the Seventh-day Adventist church.

Hospitals have conducted a variety of health education programs but in times of tight budgets it is usually the education programs for patients that get cut. There are many opportunities for health evangelism in the hospital setting but these have not been systematically developed or encouraged. Where is the evangelistic connection?

Of course, almost every hospital has at least one baptism a year resulting from someone's ministry. An occasional baptism doesn't justify the church operating a hospital. Here you have a multimillion dollar enterprise supported by hundreds of highly trained people and all you can point to is one or two baptisms a year.

Hospitals are not cost-effective health evangelism tools. Don't get me wrong, hospitals provide a lot of highly technical medical and surgical services for persons in their immediate community but a hospital's evangelistic contribution to the church is quite limited and diminishing.

There is no practical way to insert local churches or church members into the business of a hospital. A couple of hospitals in the Adventist Health System utilize local church members as community chaplains to visit and comfort the sick. Many other Adventist hospitals are reluctant to increase any affiliation with local

Seventh-day Adventist churches. They are "community" hospitals that are managed by Seventh-day Adventists. In practice, most hospitals effectively keep the church at an arms length, away from day-to-day operations.

Better Living Centers

Better living centers provide a basic level of diagnosis and treatment but their primary function is health education and rehabilitation in an institutional setting. Better living centers focus on modification of risk factors for the development of disease. The inpatient portions of these programs can last from seven to 28 days.

In the United States every better living center is self-supporting. They are not owned or operated by the Seventh-day Adventist church. These institutions are conservative in religious orientation and health practice.

Better living centers provide a vegetarian diet. Meals consist of tastefully prepared but often unfamiliar dishes. Recipes are shared and food preparation is practiced under the watchful eye of the nutrition staff.

Rigorous exercise regimens are pursued daily. These programs are adjusted for age and medical condition. Great improvements in distance and endurance are accomplished. New habits are formed.

These live-in programs often have a physical therapy component with steam baths, hot and cold contrasting showers, fomentations, and massage therapy. Soreness in the muscles is relieved.

Clients are exposed to strong spiritual influences. Every staff member freely speaks of spiritual things. There are morning and evening worship services. The Sabbath is devoted to preaching, study and conversations on spiritual topics.

The administrations of these institutions are guided by the Spirit of Prophecy counsel regarding the establishment of Sanitariums. These small institutions are also felt by many to more closely approximate what Seventh-day Adventist health institutions were meant to be, in contrast to the community hospital model.

The more well known of these better living centers are:

Weimar Institute
2061 West Paoli Lane
Weimar, CA 95736

Lifestyle Center of America
Route 1, Box 4001
Sulphur, OK 73086

Wildwood Lifestyle Center and Hospital
PO Box 129
Wildwood, GA 30757

Black Hills Health and Education Center
PO Box 19
Hermosa, SD 57744

Poland Spring Health Institute, Inc.
32 Summit Spring Road
Poland, ME 04274-6704

Eden Valley Institute
6263 N. County Road 29
Loveland, CO 80538

Uchee Pines Institute
30 Uchee Pines Road #1
Seale, AL 36875-5702

Heartland Institute of Health & Education
PO Box 1,
Rapidan, VA 22733-0001

There are other better living centers that are not as well known. The services and programs offered by each of these centers differ considerably. These institutions have been life changing and life saving to many of their clients.

Better Living Centers and the Local Church

There are fundamental problems with the better living centers. These independent ministries cannot be faulted for being separate from the administrative structure of the Seventh-day Adventist church but they are to be faulted for divorcing themselves from local Seventh-day Adventist churches.

The local church is the Christian's home not the better living center. Not one of these institutions has designed or implemented a system for creating connections between their clients and the local Seventh-day Adventist church in the home community from which the clients come. In this aspect in particular, better living centers have failed to maximize the evangelistic potential of their health programs.

The better living centers largely ignore local churches. There are some important reasons for this. Local Seventh-day Adventist churches are largely filled with intemperate people who need to know and practice the health message better than they do. Members of the local church would be a bad example to returning clients who have learned healthful living practices at the better living center. These may be the facts but do not constitute good reasons for leaving the local churches out of the picture.

Better living centers should assume the responsibility for reforming the lives of church members and help bring up the quality of life in the local church. At a minimum, better living centers should identify key members, in every church, who are living the health message. These key members would make wonderful contacts for the clients of better living centers who return home and need someone at the local level to help them maintain their new health behaviors.

Let me propose a mechanism for accomplishing this goal. Insert a local church in the process of acquiring new clients at better living centers. Instead of enrolling clients who write or call to enroll in a program at one of these sanitariums, refer all inquiries to a local Seventh-day Adventist church in the prospective client's home community.

A friendly church member, who lives in the town where the prospective client lives, can come over to their house, explain the various programs available at the better living center and show them a color brochure about the better living center. The enrollment forms can be completed by the church member who can then fax or mail them in to the central office A confirmed appointment can be communicated back to the prospective client through the local church member.

When the local church is inserted into the program of the better living center in this way, the prospective client has taken some very important evangelistic steps. He or she has met someone in their hometown who goes to the Seventh-day Adventist church. They have made a friend. This friend will help them get into the better living center but this friend will also be there when he or she comes home from the better living center.

The local Seventh-day Adventist church member can also help the client adhere to the newly acquired health habits. The church member is only a call away and should be available 24 hours a day to offer practical, moral and spiritual support.

The local Seventh-day Adventist church member can also be available to conduct periodic follow-up surveys for the better living center. This will provide the better living center with much needed long term effectiveness data that will justify the work it does. Additionally, some of the administrative burden is cast onto a volunteer system saving the better living center some money.

Setting up Local Church Affiliations

Every better living center should promote their services in local Seventh-day Adventist churches. Every weekend they should be in some church promoting healthful living. Jesus is returning to take to heaven a church that is free from every spot and wrinkle. We have too many spots and wrinkles. Too much indulgence of appetite. Too much indolence and lack of physical activity.

Every Seventh-day Adventist church within driving distance of a better living center should be visited by someone from there. Health programs should be conducted in local churches. At the same time, church members could be identified who would be willing to be affiliated with a better living center. Inventory the lifestyle of church members who volunteer for service. If found acceptable, give them some kind of credential. Perhaps a badge, a laminated card, a plaque or a letter. Give them promotional material, application forms and contact numbers for the better living center.

This should be a voluntary system. Perhaps some incentives could be built in. The church member might be able to spend a weekend now and then or participate in a short course at the better living center.

What a blessing to the local church would result from this affiliation with a better living center. Church members would live better lives and would be connected with community people who attended the live-in programs at the better living center. Church members would have a reason to call on graduates of these programs. They would regularly meet with them and help them live healthfully.

The local church can provide Bible studies to those who are interested. New church members will come from this affiliation.

Better living centers should think about good health but they should think first and foremost as to how to get people into the kingdom of God and become members of some local Seventh-day Adventist church.

Boarding Schools and Health Evangelism

Some of the better living centers have schools attached to them. Wiemar Institute has a college. Hartland Institute in Virginia has a school program as do some other institutions. In some cases these schools are recognized by the state or church but in several instances there is no accreditation. This is not especially bad. The students receive a basic education with an emphasis on healthful living and Christian principles. Much of what I have said about the local church applies to these schools as well. Many of these students have come apart from local churches that are lukewarm and lacking in evangelistic activity. These students should turn around and embrace the churches they just left and help make them evangelistic tools in their local communities.

Vegetarian Restaurants

There have been some outstandingly successful vegetarian restaurants. These institutions provide healthful food attractively prepared. These restaurants should have an educational component with literature on healthful living and classes to help people learn how to prepare healthful vegetarian meals at home.

Ways should be explored to make these institutions more evangelistic. There should be ways to tie a restaurant to a local church. Programs sponsored by the restaurant should not be conducted at the restaurant but at a local Seventh-day Adventist church. The goal of the restaurant should be to win souls for the kingdom of God and get people to worship in a local Seventh-day Adventist church.

Church Administration

Great confusion and apostasy regarding the health message have occurred at all levels of the Seventh-day Adventist church. The confusion arose in part from the former division of the health message into the Temperance and Health components. The Temperance department was concerned with tobacco, and alcohol primarily. The health department was concerned with mission hospitals and sponsored the Weigh-Rite program. At one point in time there were temperance departments at the division, union and local conference levels of church administration.

In the early 80's the Seventh-day Adventist church combined the Health and Temperance departments. This created prolonged friction and divisiveness at many levels of church administration. First Dr. Mervyn Hardinge, next Dr. Gordon Hadley and subsequently others have directed this combined Health and Temperance department at the General Conference level which is now know as the Health Ministries Department. The unified department hasn't been highly effective. At the local level we hear less and less about health evangelism each year.

Oh, yes, the Health Ministries Department has produced some material, and designed some programs but the influence of this department in the church has diminished greatly over the past 30 years. I do not believe that any union conference or local conference has a full time Health Ministries director. As a result, there is very little health and temperance activity at the local church level in the Seventh-day Adventist church today.

Adventist Community Services

Adventist Community Services is an organization dedicated to disaster relief. If there is a tornado, flood or other natural disaster, the Community Services vans are there and local church members help with distribution of clothes, blankets, and food. This is a good service which the church provides the community, but the evangelistic potential of these activities is quite small. Local church members are not encouraged to maintain any meaningful and potentially evangelistic contact with those they help.

ADRA

Adventist Development and Relief Agency, (ADRA) receives great monitory support from the church and even more from various individuals, foundations and governments around the world. ADRA handles huge amounts of money, food, clothing and relief supplies. ADRA is involved with thousands of different projects in hundreds of countries. ADRA is wonderful.

However, ADRA is not overtly evangelistic. The credit for the work ADRA does is often given to the donor organization or nation. The name Seventh-day Adventist is often not identified in the work ADRA does. By downplaying

ADRA's affiliation with the church they have gained support of the world. If your analysis of the success of ADRA is measured by effort, it is simply wonderful. If analysis of success is measured by progress toward the goals of the church, the success would be considerably less.

The church should not be involved in doing the world's relief work; particularly if the church's name is withheld in the effort. There are almost no mechanisms for connecting recipients of ADRA's help with local Seventh-day Adventist Churches. Where are the baptisms?

Less Common Church Ministries

I do not know of any night shelters operated by the Seventh-day Adventist church. In Fort Worth, the Presbyterian Night Shelter houses and feeds up to 500 people each night. This is an expensive undertaking that has the support of multiple churches and civic organizations. There are evangelistic opportunities in such a setting but I don't know to what extent they are pursued.

The Salvation Army provides shelter and food for the homeless. Their activities are combined with prayer and preaching and have been designed to be evangelistic. There is the Union Gospel Mission which is evangelistic in its efforts to help the needy. The Seventh-day Adventist church hasn't duplicated any of these service formats and may not need to.

The most available, most important and least utilized institution is the local church. It stands empty, its members occupied with the cares of the world and idle with respect to health evangelism. Let's see how to make the local church more effective in doing God's work.

Summary

1. The local church format is the least developed venue for health evangelism. There is counsel in Scripture and Spirit of Prophecy that the local church should be the focal point for soul winning activities.

2. Hospitals provide excellent care for the sick. All hospitals have chaplains to minister to the spiritual needs of patients but health evangelism has not been developed in an effective way. Only a few new church members come from hospital activities.

3. Better Living Centers have blended physical and spiritual ministries but in a vacuum. No systematic connection with local or regional churches exists. These centers aren't blessing the local churches very much.

4. Some boarding schools have a health evangelism emphasis but are lacking a connection with local churches.

5. There are a very few successful health oriented restaurants. There will always be a temptation to reduce the educational emphasis if food sells successfully.

6. Church administration has essentially abandoned health evangelism.

7. Adventist Community Services provide needed disaster relief. This helps create a good name for the church but doesn't come close to being health evangelism.

8. ADRA does a great and diverse work around the world. It is big on health but by design is small on evangelism.

4

Program Location

Health evangelism programs have been conducted in a variety of settings. In this chapter we will review the pros and cons of conducting health evangelism programs in various settings. Success depends to a large degree on the venue you choose.

My bias is toward conducting health evangelism programs in the local church. Experience has taught me that there are many advantages in using the local church building as the focal point for your medical missionary activities.

The local church building is empty and unused except for a few hours a week. The local church building is designed for group meetings. The sanctuary can be used for a large audience. Smaller health evangelism programs might be conducted in the fellowship hall, or can be held in Sabbath School rooms. So, whether you plan big or small programs, the church can hold your crowd.

The price is also right. It is your church. You shouldn't have to pay any rent to conduct a series of meetings there. Renting facilities elsewhere can be very expensive. There will be a huge cost advantage to using your own local church for health evangelism programs.

Another big advantage of conducting health evangelism programs in your local church is that the Seventh-day Adventist church will get the visibility and credit for the program. The more you do for your community in your church, the better the reputation your church will have in the community. Ideally, your church should come to the point where anyone with a problem in the community will think of your Seventh-day Adventist church as the place to go for help. This won't happen unless you begin to do something useful for your community in your church buildings.

Ownership

Ownership is a big problem with health evangelism programs. Local church members need to see that health evangelism is his or her program. Conducting health evangelism activities in the local church creates this ownership. Anything sponsored by and conducted in your local Seventh-day Adventist church is *your* program.

Health evangelism programs conducted *away* from the church will be perceived as belonging to only those few who are organizing and conducting the program. Church members will usually be neutral about such programs. To create a feeling of ownership on the part of church members the health evangelism program must be conducted in the local church.

Worse things can happen. If a health evangelism program is conducted off site, it is very likely to be perceived in a negative light. The Philadelphia Better Living Center is an example. In years past is was a centrally located health evangelism facility staffed by Dr. Vincent Gardner and his wife with the support of others.

It was supposed to be the cooperative effort of all the churches in the Philadelphia area. Programs for the public were conducted there on a regular basis. Church members from local churches provided some staff and programming support. This effort struggled and eventually failed due to lack of consistent support from local churches.

I talked with some of the local pastors about the situation and the pastors saw this health evangelism effort in a negative light. As church members became involved in the Better Living Center, they were seen less and less in the local church. It had the effect of siphoning off talent from the local church.

Pastors were unhappy because their best and most active members were dividing their time between activities in the local church and the Better Living Center. This meant a net drain on the resources of each church involved. Pastors were against it.

Here is an illustration of the ownership principle. If health evangelism programs had been conducted in local churches, the pastors might have been happier. They would see the church building used for community work. They would see non-Adventists coming to the Adventist Church on a regular basis. Pastors would see church members coming out to support "their" own programs. The pastors would have seen evangelistic possibilities.

Ownership of programs will only come about if programs are conducted in the local church with participation of local church members. You fail to establish ownership when health evangelism is conducted in other outside settings.

Church Is Nonthreatening During the Week

Conducting health evangelism programs in the local church is nonthreatening for non-church members during "off" hours. It is one thing to invite your neighbor to come to church on Sabbath or to a full set of evangelistic meetings and quite another to invite your neighbor to a cooking class or weight control program during the week.

Your neighbors don't want to come to your church if they are going to be indoctrinated but they don't mind coming to church if there is an informational or intervention program that is going to help them with a real problem. Your neighbors are much more likely to go to your church for a health program than they are to go there for spiritual services.

Neighbors are also a curious lot. While attending your health evangelism program, they will want to look the facilities over. This should be welcomed. If your program is not being conducted in the sanctuary, you should have the lights on low, perhaps the temperature adjusted to a comfortable level to encourage lingering a bit longer in the place of worship. It is nice to arrange for someone to be practicing the organ or playing the piano at the time of your meetings so that your participants can hear strains of music that will be familiar to them or at least create the comforting atmosphere expected in church.

When the time comes to invite your neighbors to church, it will work to your advantage if they have already been there, if they have sat in the pews, heard sweet music, and have looked through your hymnal until they spotted the same familiar songs they sing in their own church.

The best reason to conduct health evangelism programs in the local church is because it is the Christian's home. We are in the business of bringing people home. Let's get our neighbors and friends there as soon as possible. If they come to the church for a health evangelism program, they are almost home. If they come back time after time for a health program, they gradually become comfortable attending your church for non-Sabbath services. For these people it will be a painless transition to come back again on the Sabbath to worship with you.

So Many Churches

Churches provide an ideal location for conducting health evangelism because of the sheer numbers of churches available to use for such purposes. The Seventh-day Adventist church operates some 400 hospitals and clinics around the world. Certainly, health evangelism should be conducted in these places wherever possible.

There are probably a dozen Better Living centers in the United States, and a few more in other countries, operated by self-supporting institutions that promote health evangelism. These institutions help change lives and are evangelistic in their thrust. There are some problems with these institutions which will be addressed later. It is enough to point out that as far as numbers go, they are far too few to provide a world wide base for health evangelism.

The church operates at least 50,000 churches in 196 countries. We are growing churches faster than any other institution. Here is where health evangelism should be based. The focal point for health evangelism should be the local church. Health evangelism may be conducted elaborately in some large churches and in a more humble way in small churches but with so many churches available, it seems to me that the primary setting for health evangelism should be the local church.

This is not to say that health evangelism should never be conducted in a high school auditorium, hospital conference room or in Better Living Centers, it is just saying that all such activity will be limited in scope and influence. If we want health evangelism to reach millions, it must of necessity be conducted in local churches.

Problems Conducting Health Evangelism in the Local Church

Of course, there are disadvantages to conducting health evangelism programs in the local church. These problems are real but don't present an insurmountable barrier to the success of health evangelism. In several cases, the problems represent unique situations where health evangelism can correct the problem thus improving the situation of the local church.

One big problem has to do with the basic reputation of the SDA church in the local community. In certain instances health evangelism program would be much better attended in some public setting. In some communities there is considerable hostility against Seventh-day Adventists. Under these circumstances it would seem that conducting health evangelism programs in some other setting would be preferable to conducting programs in the local church building.

Perhaps the Seventh-day Adventist church in your community has a poor reputation because you have never consistently offered any services that the community found to be of any value. The only way to change your standing in the community is to begin to offer some service to the community that will be valued by the community.

Let's say that you offer a weight control program that is reasonably priced and is found by the participants to be effective. Additionally, this weight control program points to God as the agent of behavior change in the human life and is supported by a staff of loving church members who are genuinely interested in how you are doing. Doctrinal issues are left in the background.

If your church has a poor reputation, your first weight control program will be poorly attended. The second one will be more successful and by the third or fourth program the community will have changed its mind about your Seventh-day Adventist church. Those who attend your weight control program will recommend you to others who need help controlling their appetite.

Pretty soon, no one will want to miss out on a sure thing. Those who had negative attitudes against Seventh-day Adventists will change their mind or at least they will suspend their judgment until they have had a chance to see for themselves what kind of programs you conduct.

In my opinion, nothing will help change the standing and reputation of the Seventh-day Adventist church faster or more effectively than a health evangelism program offered frequently and consistently in the same place over and over again.

Another objection to conducting health evangelism programs in the local church has to do with the location of the church. Some churches are on back streets, off the beaten path or in an undesirable neighborhood. These undesirable features are used as an argument to conduct health evangelism programs in a more favorable location. Let me repeat that there is no more favorable location than your local Seventh-day Adventist church.

If you want to conduct only ONE health evangelism program and want to maximize the number of those who attend, you should conduct your program in the most public place possible. However; this will create a "flash-in-the-pan" type of response. There will be no lasting impact on the reputation of the local Seventh-day Adventist church.

It may be slower but it is a surer way to success if you conduct your health evangelism in the local church no matter how remote or isolated the location. It will take several programs to change your reputation in the community but the change will come. Soon the word will get out. "If you want help with (put any health problem here) go to the Seventh-day Adventist church. They really help people."

Some churches are in a physically rundown condition. You may be embarrassed by the shabby condition of your church. This makes you reluctant to conduct any public meetings there. The prospect of inviting the public to your church creates the perfect reason to fix the place up. Perhaps some siding needs replacing or the entry might need a new coat of paint. Get the carpet cleaned or replaced. God's house doesn't need to be fancy but it should be clean and neat.

The size of the church building may be a concern. You could service a larger crowd in a larger facility. Here is an error. There will be a further development of this concept later but you don't want to invite more people to your program than you can come close to. If your church is small and you only have a few members, you don't really want a large turn out to a health evangelism program.

Much of the effectiveness of health evangelism comes from the one-on-one relationships that are formed between members and the public. A large turnout in a large facility serviced by only a few church members, would defeat this purpose. The size of the facility used for health evangelism purposes should match the number of those who are available to help.

In short, small churches should plan on small programs for small groups until their numbers grow to the point where the whole church is ready to move to a larger facility. Big programs conducted by a few people that lack opportunities for one-on-one interactions have a net negative effect on the reputation of the Seventh-day Adventist church.

Some have become discouraged from conducting health evangelism programs because there are so few church members who help. Many times church members are not living up to the health message. Many churches have no health professionals to help conduct the program. At times the pastor is ambivalent about the whole thing. These issues will be discussed in the chapter on personnel.

Spirit of Prophecy Quotations on the Local Church.

The following testimonies from the pen of Ellen G. White recommended conducting health evangelism activities in every church in the land. Emphasis has been added so the key thought can be quickly identified.

Mrs. White suggests that the local church is the key institution for health evangelism. Our various institutions of higher learning have been a blessing to the church and have educated our children for useful service. We don't need more higher learning about health but more lower learning about health. People shouldn't have to go to the university to learn about healthful living, they should be able to learn how to live healthfully at church.

The Seventh-day Adventist denomination has never systematically made the local church an institution of learning for the church members. Churches should not only be institution that provides health information and services for the community but the church should be a school for church members.

The following quotation envisions a church educational effort that trains church members to provide both spiritual and health services for the community. A wide variety of activities are outlined in just a few sentences. This has never been done. Our educational institutions have never seen the local church as an extension of their campus.

Efforts in this direction could be organized by a pastor and the health professionals who are members of a local church but there would be more uniformity and consistent quality if our colleges, and universities accepted the responsibility of making local churches off campus sites where church members could receive the training suggested in this quotation.

> "*Every church* should be a training school for Christian workers. Its members should be taught how to give Bible readings, how to conduct and teach Sabbath-school classes, how best to help the poor and to care for the sick, how to work for the unconverted. There should be schools of health, cooking schools, and classes in various lines of Christian help work. There should not only be teaching, but actual work under experienced instructors. Let the teachers lead the way in working among the people, and others, uniting with them, will learn from their example. One example is worth more than many precepts." The Ministry of Healing, p. 149.

Mrs. White had a vision of the far reaching influence of health evangelism. She saw it operating from the churches in "every place" and in "every city" staffed by "church members." This plan has never been seriously considered or implemented by church administration at any level.

> "The medical missionary work is growing in importance, and claims the attention of *the churches*. It is a part of the gospel message, and must receive recognition. It is the heaven-ordained means of finding entrance to the hearts of people. It is the duty of our *church* members *in every place* to follow the instruction of the Great Teacher. The gospel message is to be preached *in every city*; for this is in accordance with the example of Christ and His disci-

ples. Medical missionaries are to seek patiently and earnestly to reach the higher classes. If this work is faithfully done, professional men will become trained evangelists." Medical Ministry, 241.

"The Lord gave me light that in *every place where a church was established,* medical missionary work was to be done. But there was in the Battle Creek church a great deal of selfishness. Those at the very heart of the work indulged their own wishes in a way that dishonored God. Dr. Kellogg was not sustained in the health reform work, the importance of which had been kept before the church for thirty years. This work was hindered because of the feelings and prejudices of some in Battle Creek who were not disposed to conform their course of action to the Lord God regarding health reform principles." Battle Creek Letters, 11.

The following quotation is very sobering because the problems created by conducting health work in venues other than the church have resulted in the very digressions from our primary purpose that were foretold. Today, health evangelism is not well organized. Health evangelism today is a strange assortment of efforts in a variety of settings. There is no unified vision. There is no consistency or clarity in the message proclaimed.

"The medical missionary work should be a part of the work of *every church in our land.* Disconnected from the church, it would soon become a strange medley of disorganized atoms. It would consume, but not produce. Instead of acting as God's helping hand to forward His truth, it would sap the life and force from the church and weaken the message. Conducted independently, it would not only consume talent and means needed in other lines, but in the very work of helping the helpless apart from the ministry of the word, it would place men where they would scoff at Bible truth." Counsels on Health, 514.

Here is a quotation that connects the sanitarium work with church-based health evangelism. Evidently, health institutions and the professional staff were to be instrumental in organizing health evangelism in local churches. Sanitariums are few in number and the modern hospitals have not done the work they should have been doing in the local church. Here is some advice Mrs. White had to a physician in a Seventh-day Adventist health institution.

"My brother, you need to call a halt. God has given you a work to do. He has honored you by placing you in the position which you now hold, and uniting with you men who will cooperate with you in the interests of that line of work for which the sanitarium was brought into existence. This institution has a work to perform as the Lord's appointed agency, and God is working with and through you. He designs that this work of health reform shall be an entering wedge, to prepare the way for the saving truth for this time, the proclamation of the third angel's message: but it is not to eclipse that message, or hinder its designed success, for then you work against truth. This message is the last warning to be given to a fallen world. The medical missionary work is to occupy its rightful place, as it ever should have done, *in every church in our land.*"Manuscript Releases Volume One, Compilation on Objectives of Our Medical Work and the College of Medical Evangelists, 235, 236.

Here is advice concerning restaurants. Restaurants were to be educational institutions. These restaurants would educate patrons about healthful eating. But even more importantly there was to be nutritional instruction given in every church and every church school. This nutritional instruction was to benefit members but was to reach beyond the church to "all our missionary fields." Here again the focus in on the local church.

"In our cities interested workers will take hold of various lines of missionary effort. Hygienic restaurants will be established. But with what carefulness should this work be done! Those working in these restaurants should be constantly experimenting, that they may learn how to prepare palatable, healthful foods. Every hygienic restaurant should be a school for the workers connected with it. In the cities this line of work may be done on a much larger scale than in smaller places. But in *every place where there is a church* and a *church school,* instruction should be given in regard to the preparation of simple health foods for the use of those who wish to live in accordance with the principles of health reform. And in all our missionary fields a similar work can be done." The Health Food Ministry, 94.

Healthful eating was to be practiced by church members and then the public was to be enlightened. This was to be done in *every church.*

"The work of combining fruits, seeds, grains, and roots into wholesome foods, is the Lord's work. In *every place where a church has been established,* let the church members walk humbly before God. Let them seek to enlighten the people with health reform principles." Counsels on Diet and Foods, 470.

Summary

The local church is an ideal location for conducting health evangelism for these reasons.

1. Doing health evangelism in the local church creates ownership of the program with the local church. This helps church members buy into this evangelistic process.

2. The church is a nonthreatening environment for the community if health evangelism programs are conducted during "off" hours when regular church services are not being conducted.

3. There are many churches in which to conduct health evangelism. There are more churches than all the schools, hospitals, clinics, restaurants and better living centers combined. There should be more health evangelism activities in churches than any other institutional setting.

4. There is strong support in the Spirit of Prophecy for conducting health evangelism in the local church setting. This is stressed over and over again in clear language.

5

Program Format

Do One Thing Well

How often should a health evangelism program be conducted? What days of the week are best? After this program what should we do next? These are all questions that have been asked by those who conduct health evangelism programs.

Many times, health evangelism programs have been scheduled to fit the desire of the program director to achieve results rapidly. At times pastors and evangelists have conducted health evangelism programs as a prelude to traditional evangelistic meetings. I have seen a 5-Day Plan to Stop Smoking attached to the front end of a 6-week evangelistic series. I have participated in evangelistic series where the first 10 minutes of an evening's presentation was a "health nugget."

Dozens of other variations have been tried by health professionals and church professionals over the decades. Very simply, none of these formats have been particularly successful or we would be still doing them today. So, what does work? How should health evangelism programs be conducted?

First, do one thing well. For reasons that are clearly stated elsewhere in this book, health evangelism programs should stand on their own. Health evangelism programs should be designed to be evangelistic in their own right. It is not particularly desirable for health evangelism programs to be directly connected to other more traditional doctrinal evangelistic programs.

In order to do one thing well, it is necessary to conduct the same health evangelism program over and over again. Not just once or twice but on a regular schedule. Not for just one year but year after year. There are many advantages of doing things this way.

Continuous programing of the same health evangelism program builds a core of dedicated church members, who become highly skilled in doing this work. They quickly learn the ropes of organization and when it is time to do the next program very little organizational effort is necessary. Everyone knows who does what and when to do it. There may be a new helper or two to orient to the program but the program runs smoothly with dedicated "permanent" volunteer staff.

Additionally, when the same health evangelism program is conducted repeatedly church members become skilled in relating to people who come for behavior change. Church members quickly learn all the excuses people offer for lack of compliance with the program. They learn the traps that befall those who are struggling with bad habits. Church members become skilled counselors.

More importantly, church members learn to pray for those who are struggling to break the bonds of sin and live better, healthier lives. They can become spiritual guides to those who need someone to place their hands in the hand of a loving Savior who helps them break bad habits.

None of these advantages can be achieved by doing a health evangelism program just once or twice and then going on to something else. Learn to do one thing well.

An additional advantage in doing just one health evangelism program is that the community will come to rely on your church for help with that particular health problem. If you conduct a weight control program, those who have been successful will advise their obese neighbors to, "Go down to the Seventh-day Adventist church. They help people with weight problems."

A good reputation is the result of consistency and reliability. We are confirmed as Seventh-day Adventists because we go to church *every* Sabbath. We will be confirmed as health evangelists if we consistently offer life saving health programing on a regular, dependable, basis.

In my community, a local Baptist church operates "Mission Fort Worth." This is a free medical clinic for the poor that operates two noon hours a week. They have been operating for years with volunteer help. They have a great reputation and offer real medical services that aren't available elsewhere. The success of this program is due to its *continuous* availability. The clinic staff also conduct home visits and Bible studies.

Other examples of ongoing health evangelism activities in Fort Worth include a dental clinic operated by the AIDS Interfaith Network. They provide dental services for the local indigent HIV/AIDS population. Another faith-based program is the Presbyterian Night Shelter.

It doesn't matter if the health evangelism effort is large, involving a complex organization and hundreds of volunteers or a simple program offered out of a church basement by a few volunteers. A program offered continuously and consistently will find a valued place in the spectrum of health services available in your community.

Another benefit of doing one program well is the networking that results. Other community agencies will start referring clients to your health evangelism program. Case workers dispensing food stamps to obese persons may advise their clients to enroll in your weight management program. And on it goes. The longer you operate the same health evangelism program in a community the more referrals you will receive from other agencies.

These other voluntary and governmental agencies will be comfortable referring clients to your health evangelism program because your program has a life of it's own and is not obviously connected with traditional evangelistic efforts. This doesn't mean you can't conduct traditional evangelistic meetings in the same church you do health evangelism but they must run on separate tracks.

Voluntary and governmental agencies will prefer to refer clients to your health evangelism programs over many other programs. Your program is a voluntary effort that is low cost. What I am saying is that the American Heart Association would rather refer an overweight client to your weight management program because you are both voluntary organizations. The Heart Association is not going to create business for Weight Watchers, Overeaters anonymous, TOPS or any for profit organization.

The national climate in the United States is such that "faith-based" initiatives are looked upon favorably. A church that offers behavior change programs of various types will be a valued community resource.

An equally important part of networking is for you to learn the services offered by other agencies in your community. You will have occasion to refer people with various needs to other organizations that can provide help to your clients.

Sequencing and Bridging

There have been many attempts to bridge the gap between health programs and evangelistic programs. Health programs have been largely secular in their design and evangelistic programs are overtly spiritual. When there is no significant spiritual emphasis in the health program the transition to evangelistic meetings is abrupt.

It was common in the 1970's for hundreds to come to the 5-Day Plan to Stop Smoking but only a few would stay for the follow-up evangelistic programs. Many minds have tried to develop a successful transition between secular and spiritual programs. Nothing has been found to work very well.

One model that was developed envisioned a whole series of programs starting with a secular program dealing with health issues followed by a psychological program dealing with stress or some other psychological issue and finally coming around to spiritual evangelistic meetings. This never worked successfully. When multiple and differing programs are all lined up in a row there will be a big drop in attendance at each transition.

If you do just one program, the audience will be composed of those who want help with the behavioral problem that program addresses. To be sure, we all have multiple problems but who is to say what we should work on next? Who are we to say that you will be best benefitted if you attend program A and then proceed to program B, followed by programs C, D and ending up with E, which stands for evangelism? I think the A-B-C-D-E approach is doomed to failure.

Don't get me wrong. I believe that many churches, especially larger ones, can offer a variety of health evangelism programs. These programs should all be on independent tracks. I illustrate the concept this way.

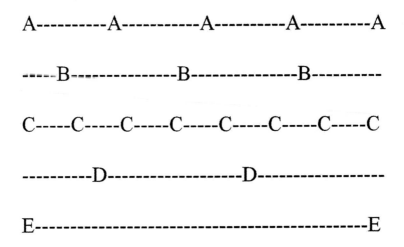

A stop smoking program should be followed by another stop smoking program. The dates for the next stop smoking program should be set before the current program is finished.

You should have the brochures printed that list all the stop smoking programs you are going to conduct for the whole year.

When a person successfully completes a smoking cessation program, he or she is MOST interested in when the next smoking cessation program is going to be held. Exsmokers have relatives and friends who need your services and they will be quick to recommend your stop smoking program to friends and associates.

Only a few who quit smoking will be interested in other programs. It is appropriate to advertise all the different programs you offer at your church in every program you conduct. All smokers who come to quit should know that there is a cooking school, a weight loss program, exercise programs and, yes, even evangelistic programs.

Some who just quit smoking will need a weight control program while others are ready to start an exercise program and a few will be ready for an evangelistic program. If you are operating continuous programing on parallel tracts the choice as to what to do next is up to the participant. No one will feel any particular pressure to attend one program or another. People like to have options. They want and appreciate the availability of choices.

Most of the time, the Holy Spirit prompts us to work on our habits sequentially. If your church offers a variety of behavioral change programs, it is likely that the Holy Spirit will prompt a person who overcame one problem to attend another one of your programs. Sequencing is an individual matter that should be under the control of the Spirit working on a person's life and not the wishes of the evangelist or health programer.

When the sequencing is A—B—C—D—Evangelism, the participant soon learns that your church doesn't offer health programs on a regular and dependable basis to serve the continuing health needs of the community but only as a prelude to traditional evangelism. I have heard evangelists repeatedly use the bait and hook analogy. The health program is the bait and the doctrinal presentations are the hooks.

I reject this analogy and the entire thought process behind it. I feel that health programs should be evangelistic in and of themselves. Participants who are enslaved by some life destroying habit should be pointed to Jesus as the agent of real and lasting change in the human life. Health evangelism, rightly conducted is the bait AND the hook. Let me emphasize this by asking, "If a person's life wasn't changed by God in your health program why should they have any interest in your doctrinal discussions?" However, those who have had a taste of God's power in their lives as they overcome a bad habit, are those who will hunger and thirst for more. This thought is more fully developed in another chapter.

Duration of a Program

How long should a health evangelism program run? How many times a week should you meet? The 5-Day Plan to Stop Smoking was great because it ran five days and was over with. You could wedge it in between weekends. There was a one week investment of time and then you were through.

It would have been nice to study the optimum time required to achieve lasting success when quitting smoking and then design a program to fit the needs of the smokers who wanted to quit. The ideal duration of a smoking cessation program hasn't been determined exactly. I have observed smoking cessation programs of varying duration. On the short side, I have seen an all-day-long, 8-12 hour, marathon smoking cessation program. The hope was, that you could quit smoking in just one day. On the long end, there is SmokeEnders, a program that lasts several weeks. What is best?

There are several issues to consider in determining the duration of a health evangelism program. Perhaps most important is, how long can you run a program that people will still attend. We would like to think that the public is very interested in health information and is willing to spend as much time as necessary to be properly educated and to get one's habits changed.

This just isn't true. Some programs need to be nightly for a few nights. I believe that smoking cessation fits in this category. The cravings are intense for just a few days and attending meetings every day can keep you from relapsing. Other programs should be drawn out and conducted at a slower pace over a much longer period of time.

For many health evangelism programs, conducting meetings just once a week is ideal. The less frequent the meetings, the longer the program will need to run. Don't over do it. I have seen intense nutrition programs run four nights a week for a month. The material presented was excellent and the speaker was captivating but it was an overload for the public and for the church members who really didn't support the program as well as they should have. This particular program might have been better supported by the public and local church members if it ran one night a week for three or four months rather than 16 sessions crammed into just one month. Some churches offer a health program just one session per month but keep it up on a year around basis.

After you decide what is best for the participants who are going to come to your program it is best to consult with your church members and determine just how much time they are willing to devote to your program. If you plan to have small groups hosted by church members, it is important to find out just how often church members are willing to meet and for how many weeks. In my experience, you get the most help from individual church members when the program is offered on a one night a week basis. If you conduct the same program with the same volunteers two or three nights a week, the help will be strained and will begin to drop out or fail to volunteer for your next program

As a general rule, it is wise to avoid weekend days and nights for a lot of programs unless you have a one session program such as a health fair, in which case a weekend day might work out well.

Summary

The success of a program with the community and church members will depend on several factors.

1. Do one thing well. Do one thing over and over again until church members become skilled in organizing, conducting and following up a health evangelism program.

2. Sequencing to some other type of health program will kill the program you are doing successfully right now.

3. Trying to create a bridge between health evangelism and traditional evangelism will hurt your program.

4. Developing additional health evangelism programs in a local church is wise only after you have learned to do one thing well. Your new program should not replace your original program but just be another parallel service of your church.

5. Conduct traditional evangelistic efforts at regular times. Invite all who are currently in or who have ever attended health evangelism programs in the past to attend. Programs promoting distinctive doctrines are necessary and expected but run on a separate track. All are welcome but traditional evangelism is a separate activity of the church.

6

Organizing a Health Evangelism Program

Groundwork

Talk up health evangelism and see what happens. Explore health evangelism with the pastor of the church. Has the pastor ever conducted or participated in a health evangelism program? When was the last time? What role did the pastor have? What was the result? Was the experience positive or negative? Would the pastoral staff be interested in having a health evangelism program in the present location? Would he or she help by giving a talk each night of the program? Would the pastor help promote the program in the church? The answers to all of these questions are important before beginning to promote your health evangelism program.

Next, it is important to feel out some of the church leaders to see if they would be supportive and to find out if they would participate. Have a chat with the head elder, head deacon and deaconess. Find out if there are any health professionals in the church. Have any of them ever taken part in a health evangelism program? Are they willing to help? Will they be able to give one or more talks during the program?

Lastly, and I don't put as much emphasis on this as many do, find out what will be received favorably by the community. Some go to great lengths to do a "needs assessment" of the community. That is fine, but I can tell you that if you do a door-to-door survey you will find smokers, sedentary people, overweight people, alcoholics and people who need stress reduction.

If you have the time to do a community survey, please be my guest, but I don't look upon surveys as particularly important. Pick an established health evangelism program or design one of your own and offer it to the public. Your advertising and the Holy Spirit will bring to your program just those who need your help.

After conducting the same program over and over a few times, your reputation will be such that no further advertising will be necessary and all your meetings will be crowded. Just choose something, get started and do it. The public will come.

Announcing the Health Evangelism Program to the Church

It is usually most effective in getting church member attention and cooperation if the announcement of the organization of a health evangelism program is made at church during the church service. It is useful if the sermon focuses on service, individual responsibility and a call to church members to commit themselves to the health evangelism program you have chosen to conduct in that church.

At the end of the sermon a call should be made, a show of hands, for those who are willing and planning to support the upcoming health evangelism program. At the same time, the first organizational meeting including time and place, should be announced and all who raised their hands should be encouraged to come.

Now begins what I call the "Gideon process." Of all those who raised their hands at church, only a small fraction will show up for the first organizational meeting. Once the details of the program are laid out at the organizational meeting, only a few will find that the health evangelism program will fit into their schedule. As preparation continues from week to week, before your program actually begins, additional church members will drop out but at times others can be recruited to fill special positions.

Do not be discouraged by the attrition of church members. It is much better to lose these faint-of-heart or too busy folk from your program before it starts than to lose them during the program. Loss of church members during the program is tragic. It leaves gaps in coverage of small groups and creates the impression of disorganization and even a "not caring" attitude on the part of the church.

The First Organizational Meeting

Order is the first law of Heaven. Any task undertaken by the church should be appropriately organized with a careful distribution of labor. At the first organizational meeting about half the time should be spent in spiritual preparation. You should give a short spiritual talk, perhaps relating to behavior change. This should be followed by a season of prayer. The last half of the meeting can be spent in an overview of the proposed program. This is where you get down to the "nuts and bolts" details.

This should include possible dates for the program and a detailed listing of all the job descriptions and an overview of how the program will run. It is good to have the first organizational meeting on the same night you plan or propose to conduct your health evangelism program. If people have trouble coming to the organizational meetings because of a conflict in schedules it is a sure thing they won't make the regular meetings either.

Do not be surprised at the small turn out at the first organizational meeting. After reviewing all the job descriptions and an outline of the time commitment that will be required in order to do the program well, there will be others that don't feel they have the time or interest to make a commitment of the magnitude required to be fully supportive.

At the first organizational meeting the dates for starting your health evangelism program should be determined. Make some preliminary plans for advertising. It would be good to organize small groups, lining up as many group leaders (partners) as possible. This will give you and the helpers an idea of how many participants should be registered for the program. If ten small group partners are identified then registration should be limited to the first 30-36 interests who call.

I like to have people preregister by calling in their reservations. If the response is poor, additional advertising can be done before the program begins to try and recruit additional participants so as to round out the program. After two or three identical health evangelism programs have been conducted, little if any advertising will be necessary as word of mouth from previous participants will quickly fill all available slots.

The most important part of preparing church members is their own spiritual preparation. I like to have church members read an appropriate passage in the Spirit of Prophecy before coming to each training session. My favorite first assignment is the chapter, "In Contact With Others" from Ministry of Healing pages 483-496. Reading assignments for church members include the following.

1.   "In Contact With Others," Ministry of Healing 483-496.

2.   "Helping the Tempted," Ministry of Healing 161-169.

3.   "Working for the Intemperate" Ministry of Healing 171-182.

4.   "Help in Daily Living" Ministry of Healing 469-482.

5.   "He Ordained Twelve" Desire of Ages 290-297.

6.   "Give Ye Them to eat" Desire of Ages 364-371.

7.   "The First Evangelists" Desire of Ages 349-358.

8.   "Duty to Preserve Health" Counsels on Health. 563, 566.

9.   "True Motive in Service" Mount of Blessing, 79, 101.

10. "Medical Evangelism" Counsels on Health 503-508.

11. "Religion and Health" Counsels on Health 28-31.

There are hundreds of texts from the Holy Bible that can be assigned for study as well.

These reading assignments are not designed to provide technical or scientific training for the church members. These are passages that spiritually prepare the church member for ministry. In each training session at least half of the preparation time should be spent in spiritual preparation of the church members.

Church members usually have better health habits than those who are coming for help. Church members quite naturally have a superiority complex about their own lifestyle and tend to be critical and unforgiving of those who are seeking help.

In order to become empathetic it is helpful to ask church members to read the assigned passage and to identify and share with the group that portion of their reading that gave them the most *instruction* or *correction*. It is heart warming to see church members confess their hard heartedness and unforgiving attitude as these defects are identified in the reading they do.

Prayer is important in preparation. Prayer should be made for the Holy Spirit to identify people in the community who particularly need your health program. The Holy Spirit can bring your advertising to their attention. The Holy Spirit creates within the mind and heart a sincere desire to change. The Holy Spirit will bring to your program just those who will be benefitted by what you are offering.

Prayer also prepares the members to participate in the program. Prayer gives your helpers a burden for souls. It creates a desire to be of service. Prayer softens the words and attitudes. Prayer makes your helpers the attractive, loving assistants your audience will need.

Pray for each other. Pray for the church. Pray for those who need to come. Pray for those who are coming. Prayer prepares the members and prepares the pubic to attend.

After the spiritual preparation of your church members it is time for job assignments. I list all of the jobs that are needed to do the program effectively. Each job description should be presented and discussed. Church members who feel they can do a specific job can volunteer. Keep track of who volunteers for what.

Gradually, the roster of jobs is filled. In a large church some larger jobs can be further subdivided so everyone will have something to do. In smaller churches or in a large church where only a small number of members volunteer, it may be necessary for one church member to do several jobs.

It will usually take three to fours weeks of preparation to get all jobs assigned and a team to be built. I want to reemphasize that about half the preparation session should be spent in spiritual preparation and half the time dividing up the various jobs. With careful preparation, when the program begins, you will have a united group of helpers who will be anxious to help those who come for help.

Church Members and Small Groups

The key element of every health evangelism program should be small groups. No matter who developed the program you are using and no matter how it was designed to be conducted, it is important to modify the program so that participants spend a substantial amount of time in small groups, teamed with partners from the congregation.

Small group activities should take from one third to one half of your program time. It is in small groups that specific problems are identified. It is in small groups that victories are shared. It is in small groups that the success of the program is realized.

Small groups should be led by church members. There should be a minimum of two church members assigned to each small group. It is also important to limit the number of participants in each small group. I like to keep the ratio of church members to small group members quite small. Ideally not more than 1:3. With two partners for each small group that allows for a total of about six participants in each small group. With the two leaders, that is eight people total in each small group.

This feature of health evangelism is so important that I limit the number of community participants based on the number of small group partners I have been able to recruit for a particular program. If I had five small groups led by 10 church members, I would then limit enrollment for this session to 30-36 community participants.

If there were many more people who wanted to come to our health evangelism program we would take their names and numbers and use the overflow as the nucleus for our next program, but I would *not* enlarge the number in each group to accommodate all who were interested in attending the program.

The purpose of small groups is to create an environment where intimate sharing can occur. The bigger the group the poorer the group dynamic. We should only invite or allow as many participants to come to a program as we have the personnel necessary to give them personal attention.

I doubt the long term effectiveness of huge health evangelism programs conducted by skilled and highly educated health professionals. I am sure the speakers appreciate the applause they get, but where is the personal, individual contact?

The interface with the public participant should be the church member who in many cases has the same weaknesses and struggles. The health professional should be available to answer technical questions but real friendships are formed in the small groups between church members and participants who come from the community.

In asking for volunteers to be small group partners it is important to keep follow-up activities in mind and to make sure church members know that their services are needed every day of the program and also after the program to conduct an adequate and complete follow-up. Follow-up will take as much time as conducting the program. Follow-up should continue at quarterly intervals for a whole year.

Materials

This is a list of the materials and documents you should obtain or develop yourself in order to be able to conduct a health evangelism program properly. If time is taken to carefully develop materials that aren't commercially available, it will greatly simplify conducting future programs. These materials will be useful if you export your health evangelism program to other churches in your area.

1. Director's Manual.

    a. Description and overview of the program and it's organization.

    b. Job descriptions

     c.   Spiritual assignments

     d.   Advertising pieces

2. Partner's Guide

3. Participants Workbook

4. Data Management

5. Educational handouts.

6. Other materials

Director's Manual

If you aren't fortunate enough to get one with the program you are conducting it will be useful to make up one as you go along. It should have documentation of everything you do. It should contain samples of all the material you need to conduct a program

The director's manual will contain a job description for every activity involved in the program. This will give the program director the overview of how to organize and conduct the program. The job description for each specific task should be copied and distributed to each church member who volunteers for each job. With written job descriptions, there will be no confusion about who has which assignment and exactly what the requirements of that assignment are. If the program you are conducting doesn't have job descriptions, it would be good to compose them and write them down during the organizational meetings.

The director's manual will have all the spiritual assignments that are to be made. I leave it to you to select appropriate scripture lessons to be assigned. Selections from the Spirit of Prophecy have been suggested above.

The director's manual should contain a copy of all the advertising pieces you developed to promote your program. Keep copies of letters sent to doctors offices, articles written for the local papers, advertising you put in local papers, scripts used on the radio or TV and form letters you sent to participants who took part in other programs. Copies of posters, banners, brochures, and handouts should be catalogued and kept in the directors manual. This will be helpful when you repeat the program. A directors manual will help others who want to do your program in their own church.

The director's manual should contain a copy of the Partner's Guide, Participants Workbook, data management pieces, educational handouts, multimedia presentations and any other materials that are used in conducting your program.

Partner's Guide

The Partner's Guide is a manual used by the helpers in your program. I like to call the helpers "Partners." Using the term "Coach" implies someone who knows more about the problem than you do and who isn't really in the struggle with you. A coach urges you on but stands on the sidelines.

The church members who are helpers are obviously mentors and group leaders but the term "partner" suggests a coequal struggling. I don't use the words: counselor, adviser, instructor, guide, mentor or group leader as they imply a position of superiority. It may be true that your partners are healthier, smarter and closer to God than many who come for help but it is never good to have a superiority complex when doing health evangelism. The term "partner" implies that you are in this together. You are going to work on the problem as a team and stick with it until the job is done.

The Partner's Guide will contain all the materials the partner will need to conduct the small groups. It will include a copy of the Participant's Workbook because they will need to lead the discussion in small groups and help the participants complete the workbook assignments.

The Partner's Guide will contain little in the way of additional educational material. If the partner heard the lecture, they will know pretty much all they need to know to help the participants with the exercises that are provided in the participant's Workbook.

What is particularly helpful to include in the Partner's Guide is material on conducting small groups. Include material on being a good listener and how to be an effective facilitator in small groups. Describe how to lead discussions. Include tips on how to channel the energies of the outspoken group members and how to draw out discussion from quieter group members.

The Partners Guide should include personal information about the members of the group. Start with a list of each of the participants in the group with their addresses and phone numbers. I encourage partners and participants to keep in touch with each other during the interval between meetings.

Find out what times are best to call participants. Is it ok to call them at work or should they wait until a participant gets home after work? Give each participant your phone numbers and indicate the best times for them to call you. Participants should be encouraged to initiate phone calls but if a group leader doesn't hear from a participant for several days it is appropriate to call and see how things are going.

If the relationship progresses beyond phone calls then so much the better. In every group there will be special friendships formed. Sometimes a participant and a group leader will share a common hobby or interest and they will make time to visit with one another and share experiences. They may meet for lunch at a restaurant or at one another's houses.

In one 5-Day Plan I conducted, a smoker was linked with a church member, George. They had been assigned to each other by the person registering people at the beginning of the program. As they got to know each other the first night of the program, they found that they worked in the same building but on different floors.

What a help George was to that smoker who was trying to quit. George and the smoker would eat lunch together. They would walk around the building to get some fresh air. George was called several times a day when the ex-smoker would have a craving for a cigarette. In short order these two were special friends.

Participants Workbook

The Participant's Workbook can be just an empty folder with pockets to keep handout materials as they are provided from session to session during the program. If there are going to be a lot of handouts it will be better to provide inexpensive three ring notebooks in which to keep material. Be sure to 3-hole punch your handouts before the program so they will fit into the notebook without additional fuss on the part of the participants.

The handouts that go into the Workbook would include copies of the health lectures, copies of all supplemental materials that are used during the program and the questionnaires and exercises that are conducted in small groups. Keep progress records in the workbook as well. Weight loss charts should be kept there for reference in a weight management program.

Data Management

So many health evangelism programs are lacking in documentation of their effectiveness. If you don't keep statistics on what happened in your program you only have the vaguest idea of what really went on. Almost every church has someone who is into computers. Get them to help you with data collection and data processing.

To start with, the program director needs a list of all the volunteers who are helping with this program. This should include names, numbers and the jobs for which they volunteered. Next is the all-important registration form. It should contain basic demographic data on those who register for your program. This should include name, address, phone numbers, sex, marital status and age.

The registration form then needs to ask questions about the behavior the participant is trying to change. For a weight control program it would be nice to know the person's current weight, maximum weight, the most they had ever lost by dieting, any health problems and whether or not they thought God would help them lose weight or if that was a problem they would have to handle by themselves.

You might ask about specific behaviors that contribute to obesity such as the number of meals eaten in a day. Get information about snack habits, about deserts, soda consumption, and alcohol consumption. The registration form might ask questions about a persons knowledge about certain nutritional principles. You could measure attitudes about weight loss etc. This is not only a registration form but an intake questionnaire that will document a person's "before" behaviors and attitudes.

It is good to measure what happened during the program by administering an exit questionnaire the last night of the program. In this questionnaire you want to ask for feedback about various elements of the program. The location isn't going to change but you could ask about the duration of the program, the quality of the speakers, the helpfulness of the small groups and any suggestions for change they might have.

The beauty of keeping statistics is that it gives you a good excuse to call on your participants after the program is over. You are wanting to measure the long term effectiveness of your program so you can make improvements in future programs. You tell your audience that you will be calling on them to obtain this information quarterly for one year after the end of the program. You are going to visit with them in their homes, in the name of scientific inquiry, to determine their progress and to help with any problems that have come up in the meantime.

All of this data is entered into a database in your computer. You can generate letters inviting your participants to other programs and of course, you will notify them when the next program they attended will be offered so they can invite their friends.

Internet web-based, software is being developed that will allow local churches to register this database information online in a confidential manner. This will simplify data collection and analysis.

Summary

Organizing and conducting a health evangelism program should be a thoughtful and careful process that include these steps.

1. Ground work with the pastor to make sure there is sympathy and support.

2. Groundwork with the church board and officers.

3. Presentation to the church as a whole to seek support. You want people to volunteer to do the work.

4. Organizational meetings will identify the sincere helpers.

5. Materials need to be acquired or developed for the director of the program, each helper and each participant who comes to change behavior.

6. Data collection and management will document what you have done. This will be useful in promoting your programs in other settings.

7

Conducting a Health Evangelism Program

You have decided to conduct a health evangelism program. You have promoted it in the church, recruited volunteers, and organized everyone and everything. Now it is opening night. Time to conduct your program.

The following program format has worked best for me. I have used it for cooking schools, weight control programs, smoking cessation programs and exercise programs. Your program should contain the following program elements.

Registration

On the first night of the program have all your staff at the church an hour early. This will allow for early completion of the set-up. It is important to be ready to roll when the first participants show up. On the first night, a few individuals usually show up 30-45 minutes before the program starts and it looks better if everything is in place long before the program begins.

Ideally, on the first night, you can have greeters out in the parking lot to assure participants that they are in the right place. Attendants can help with the parking. Attendants can point to the right door to enter. If the parking lot isn't well-lit, they should have flashlights to provide some light.

Greeters should be at the front door to warmly welcome people. They should use the name of the program repeatedly so participants will be reassured that they are at the right place. Signs or posters about the program should be placed in the lobby and at registration tables to provide additional reassurance that the participants are in the right place.

Register people in the lobby. There should be one table where people pay for the program, if a charge is made. Some health evangelists never charge for any program they conduct. I find no fault with this. On the other hand, paying something to attend a program helps establish it's value and credibility with the people.

At times, skeptical or wary participants, before they lay out any money, will want to attend a session or two to see for themselves whether or not this is a program they want to attend. They will ask if this is acceptable and promise to pay later. You should always agree to this. The object of the program is to help people—not to make money. It is also wise to have a group or family discount package. This will encourage friends and family to come together. They will think they have a real bargain if two can get in for the price of one or three can get in for the price of two.

After collecting the registration fee, give each participant the registration form and intake questionnaire. Point them to the tables set up in the lobby and ask them to sit down and fill out the forms. Have pencils and pens at every table and enough tables set up to handle the expected crowd. It will take longer than you think for them to complete the paperwork.

If anyone questions the need for you to know the information requested on your form, you can instruct them to leave blank the parts they are uncomfortable with. You can tell them that all participants are a part of a scientific study to evaluate the effectiveness of this particular program and the information will be kept confidential and only used to tabulate trends and measure effectiveness.

It avoids a lot of confusion later if small groups are formed right at the time of registration. It is good to have a separate sheet of lined paper for each small group laid out on the registration table. As a participant turns in his or her completed registration form, their name is written on a sheet belonging to one of the groups. The participant should also be given their group number. You might write it at the top of the participant's workbook.

It is appropriate for husband and wife to be assigned to the same group if they wish. Groups of friends might all want to be put in one group as well. With a glance at the group composition papers you will be able to know how many are in each group. You can make adjustments to group size as the people register. This will even out group size so they will all remain about equal.

At registration you should hand out the Participant's Workbook. It will be empty except for the first night's handouts, and worksheets. Or, you can just hand out an empty folder and tell the participants that they will receive handouts in their small group. Have their small group number written on the workbook so they will know where to go when you break out into small groups.

Give everyone a name tag to wear. These tags will be useful in small groups. Those conducting the program should wear name tags as well. Participants should wear their tags for a couple of weeks. By then they will know everyone in their small groups and name tags are less important. I prefer that all the church members who are helping in the program should wear their name tags every night for the entire program.

Next you direct the participants to the room where the program is to be held. You may hold small programs in a Sabbath School class room. A fellowship hall is good for larger programs. I think it is appropriate to use the sanctuary for health evangelism programs if it is the best room for the size of crowd you have.

Any PA system or Audio-visual equipment should be set-up long before the first participant comes into the auditorium to sit down. It is appropriate to have some classical or light music playing. It breaks the silence before the program begins and provides a cover for whispered conversations which will occur during the wait.

Welcome

Once everyone is in their places, it is time for the health evangelism program to begin. The master of ceremonies should stride purposefully to the podium and stand there until he or she has everyone's attention. In a strong voice he or she should welcome everyone to the evening's program. The master of ceremonies should repeat the name of the program several times during his remarks. This will again reassure everyone that they are in the right place.

I like to have one of the church members be the master of ceremonies. A church member usually works out better than a minister or the health professional. A church member can also talk up the program without it appearing like boasting.

During the welcoming remarks there should be laid out for the audience the whole outline of what is going to take place during the evening. This will let people know what is coming and just what they can expect. It is also good to outline the entire program. Remind them of how long the program will last in terms of weeks and what time you expect to dismiss each night. On the first night point out the location of restrooms.

Now it is time for the introductions. Introduce the health professionals who are there and mention the parts they will take in the program. Introduce the pastor. Introduce the small group concept and point out the tables or rooms where the small groups will meet. Have the partners stand so they can see just how many people are working together to bring this program to them.

Acknowledge the help of all who had a part in putting the program on. In this way the audience will see that this isn't a commercial program put on by one or two individuals for the purpose of financial gain but a group effort of a substantial number of church members. Reinforce the concept that all the workers are volunteers. This program is an effort of love for the community.

It would be good to reassure those who paid a registration fee that the funds raised do not go to support the local church. Church members are volunteers. The funds raised support community programing at various levels and to purchase materials necessary to conduct the program. It should be stressed that NO ONE is being compensated in any way for participating in the program. All are volunteers. This will raise the credibility of what you are doing in the eyes of the audience.

The Health Lecture

Introduce the first speaker and get started. Although, we don't want to boast or conduct programs in our own strength it is important for the public to know that your health evangelism program is credible and is conducted by qualified individuals. At each introduction take time to briefly state the professional qualifications of your various speakers and their experience.

The first speaker should present the medical or scientific portion of your program. It might be a medical doctor speaking about lung disease, cancer, or heart disease at a smoking cessation program. It might be a dietician at a weight control program or cooking school. As far as possible use help available in your own congregation.

If there are no health professionals in your church, the presentations can be done by lay persons who have studied up on the topic and can speak with some confidence. For one or more sessions you might invite a health professional who is not a member of your church to speak. It should be someone who has respect in the community and one whom you know is sympathetic to the objectives of your program.

The Pastor's Part

Next, I like to have the pastor speak about behavior change. Introduce the pastor as the pastor of the church. It is appropriate to indicate when he preaches and invite any who wants to, to come to regular church services. I find it effective if the master of ceremonies comes back up between each part of the program and announces what is going to happen next. Also, since the health professional was introduced with an emphasis on what he or she does, it is appropriate to have the pastor introduced and mention the pastor's qualifications and pastoral services available at the church.

I have been to health evangelism programs where the pastor spoke and managed to squeeze in three or four of the distinctive doctrines of the Seventh-day Adventist church in during the course of his talk. This is just wrong. Your health evangelism program is about behavior changes needed to improve health not distinctive doctrines. The health evangelism program is problem specific evangelism not broad spectrum evangelism. The pastor should stick to behavior change from a Christian/Biblical perspective.

There are many books on psychology describing the steps involved in behavior change. The principles in these books correctly describe the mental and behavior steps one goes through in changing behavior but these books don't have the ability to impart the POWER to accomplish behavior change. Lasting behavior change comes from God. The pastor knows God and should speak to how God helps people bring about lasting change in their lives.

Will people be offended by this? Some will, but most won't. If the pastor focuses on how God helps with the specific problem at hand, no one will leave the program. Most of your participants are desperate people. They have tried to change their behaviors many times, on their own, in the past and have failed. Frankly, they are willing to listen to any angle (including God's help) if there is even a remote chance that it will work for them now.

If participants object to the spiritual material in the program, offer to refund their registration fee and wish them well. They will continue to search for help outside of the help that God offers. Over the years, many different health evangelism programs have been developed by health educators in the Seventh-day Adventist church. Many of these programs have left God's help out of their lecture material. In failing to point to God as the agent of behavior change, these programs failed to be evangelistic and were just health programs.

In most communities there are many Godless self-help programs. If a participant at your weight control program is offended that you suggest that God will help them lose weight, let them go to Weight Watchers, TOPS, Overeaters Anonymous, Jenny Craig or a dozen other weight control programs. If a participant at your smoking cessation program is offended that you point to God as the One who can help them overcome the addiction to smoking, refer them to the American Cancer Society, American Heart Association, The American Lung

Association, local hospital, or health insurance company where they can receive help in quitting smoking the Godless way.

Where is the addict to learn that God will help them? They should learn this at a Seventh-day Adventist church. We hate to see anyone turn away from the church to seek help elsewhere, but, there are hundreds of Godless, self-help programs for these people to go to and enroll in. Where are the programs that point to God as the Help for human helplessness? Health evangelism programs that introduce people to God as the helper for every problem should be found in every Seventh-day Adventist church in the world.

If the pastor is supportive of your health evangelism program but unable or unwilling to speak on behavior change, others can be chosen to do this part. This behavior change through God's help is the evangelistic key to success in your program. It should not be omitted under any circumstances. This emphasis is effective coming from a health professional or any layperson who has experienced God's help in overcoming some habit.

Demonstrations

If your health evangelism program has demonstrations, this is a good time in the program to do them. Food demonstrations are useful in weight management programs and essential in cooking schools. Smoking Sam is a useful demonstration at smoking cessation programs. Showing the correct type of clothing and shoes for an exercise class are appropriate.

Small Groups

I like to end the program with small group activity. At least 1/3 of the time for the session should be spent in small groups. At the first session, when it is time for small groups, it is best to have the partners stand and hold up numbers for the group they are going to facilitate. If the tables are in the same room as the lecture they can be clearly labeled so there is no confusion about where each group is to meet.

If you are utilizing rooms elsewhere in your church for small groups, those rooms should be clearly marked and maps should be distributed so it will be easy for everyone to find their way to their assigned group. Partners should be dismissed first so they can lead the way to their locations and be there to welcome group members as they come in.

At the first session, each group leader should have a copy of the small group composition forms that were developed during registration. This will tell the small group partners how many to expect in their group and the names of those who are coming. There may be some shifting of group composition on the first night as people who come meet others they know and want to shift groups to be with acquaintances. All this shifting is acceptable and adjustments in the lists need to be made so the composition of each group is accurately known.

In the small group everyone should have name tags. The first order of business is introductions all around. Exchange names, background, interests and hobbies. The object is to make the group feel comfortable, to break the ice, and to give a feeling of informality.

Goals are good to discuss. What is each person wanting to get out of this program? What have they tried before? How far did they get in previous trials? Try to be as specific as possible. In a weight control program, ask how much weight does the participant want to lose during the 10 weeks of the program? These goals are written down in the participant's workbook.

In the small group the main discussion should center around the suggested behavior changes spoken of in the evening's lecture. For instance, if the health professional suggested eating less sugar, the small group members would discuss where the most sugar is in their diet. Once the source of excess sugar is identified, each small group member should make a specific commitment to reduce their sugar intake during the coming week.

For one, it might be the elimination of sodas or switching to diet sodas. For another it might be eating fewer deserts—perhaps limiting deserts to just one serving a week. In the small group you individualize the prescription that was given in a general way in the lecture.

You can develop additional handouts on the subject of the night. This material can be read in a leisurely manner at home. Some nights there can be a quiz over the evening's topic. Once everyone has completed the quiz, the partners can provide the answers and this can be the focal point of additional discussion.

The partners should offer their availability to help with any problems that might come up during the interval between programs. They should distribute their day and evening phone numbers and indicate the best times to be called. Participants should be responsible for calling their partners if they are having problems. It is also appropriate for partners to contact their members at least once during the week just to keep tabs on them and to encourage them to come back to the next session.

Partners will sometimes have occasion for further socialization with group members outside of small group time at the church. All this activity should be encouraged. Church members have been known to go shopping with group members. Others have met after work and gone to a restaurant together. The options for socialization are unlimited. Lasting friendships are formed from these informal contacts.

This is the interface the church needs with its community; church members becoming friends with non-church members. This will have more to do with evangelism than any preaching will do. Most people join the church because they have friends in the church. Small groups are where these friendships are formed.

The health professional and pastor should remain for small groups. They should not join a small group or dominate a small group but should be available to clarify points and answer specific questions that may be beyond the scope of knowledge of the small group leader. Knowing this additional help is available will encourage many church members to volunteer as small group partners because they will never be stuck. Someone will always be available to help them should the need arise.

Small group partners don't have to be experts. Their role is to facilitate discussion. The topic is the evening's lectures. There are handouts that cover the topic further and a questionnaire facilitates discussion. Be sure the partners have the answers to any quizzes you use along with an explanation of the answers.

Dismiss the program for the night from the small groups. Groups will break up at slightly different times and the evening's program will gradually dissolve away.

After Glow (Post Program Assessment)

Immediately after the last small group has been dismissed, call all the helpers and small group partners together for an assessment of the evening's program. There are several tasks to take care of.

Review activities that occurred in small groups. There will be stories of victory and overcoming which will cheer the hearts of all and should be shared. There will be special problems that certain participants are having. These difficulties should be recognized and special efforts made to help those participants who are struggling.

There should be a short season of prayer. Thank God for the success and the opportunity to witness and ask for God's special blessing on those who are wrestling with addictions and bad habits.

There should be an accounting of those participants who did not attend the evening's meeting. Some will have valid reasons for not attending while others will just not be accounted for. The small group partners should take the responsibility of contacting their own members who did not attend and find out what the problem was.

If absent participants are not planning on coming back they should be let go without too much fuss. It will be useful to see if they want to be notified of future programs; if so, retain them on your mailing list. If they aren't interested in any further contact with your church, it is the courteous thing to do to remove their names from your mailing list.

This entire "after glow" process should be limited to about 15 minutes. Your helpers/partners will be anxious to get home and prolonging this session will discourage future participation if carried on too long.

Summary

There are many ways to conduct a program. You may arrange the component parts in a way to best suit your circumstances. A general outline for conducting a program that has worked well for me is summarized below.

1. Registration. Collecting fees. Assignment to small groups.

2. Welcome by the master of ceremonies. Explanation of the program flow and introduction of the various speakers as well as small group partners.

3. Health lecture.

4. Pastor's part.

5. Demonstrations of various type in some programs. How to make certain dishes etc.

6. Small groups. About a third to a half of the time should be spent in small groups. Two church members lead a discussion with 6-8 community members who are taking part in the program.

7. After glow. This is a time to review successes and problems that came up in the program.

8

Finding the Right Personnel

Who are the people who should be conducting health evangelism programs? What is the personnel mix you need for a successful program? The 5-Day Plan to Stop Smoking was conducted by a doctor and minister team. In some places these programs were conducted by other health professionals and even by laymen. Let's look at personnel issues in conducting health evangelism programs.

The Minister

It is natural to assume that a health evangelism program conducted in the local church should utilize the services of the local pastor. Yes, there is a role for your pastor in health evangelism, but I believe the pastor's role should not be central to the program. The role of the pastor in health evangelism programs needs careful discussion.

The pastor should be visible and acknowledged as the pastor in every health evangelism program. I believe the pastor should have something to say, even if it is just a word of welcome, at every meeting. The pastor may present a major topic on some nights of the program but at other times be just a quiet presence.

The pastor is a busy person. It is NOT necessary or desirable for the pastor to personally conduct every program at the church. Health evangelism programs should be conducted by church members. Pastors have many responsibilities including, visitation, Bible studies, counseling and a host of other activities that occupy their time. If your pastor is particularly busy but generally supportive of health evangelism programs, give your pastor a break and structure your health evangelism program so the pastor has only token involvement.

Over the course of years, pastors tend to come and go. If health evangelism programs are too dependent on the pastor an established program might just die if the pastor moved away. It is better to have health evangelism programs established, conducted and maintained by church members. In this way there will be more stability if the pastor moves on to other assignments.

Then again, some pastors don't live the health message. Pastors who are overweight, don't exercise regularly, openly drink coffee or tea will tend to have a negative influence on the health evangelism programs you conduct. Under these circumstances, it might be wise not to conduct any health evangelism programs in your church until the situation is more favorable.

At times, pastors become jealous of the success church members are having in doing health evangelism programs. When this occurs a subtle antagonism will develop toward you, your committee or the health evangelism program itself. The pastor may consistently come to your program late or boycott a meeting or two. The pastor may suggest interrupting an established cycle of health evangelism programs so he may conduct some other program he is more interested in. If this should happen to you, it will be better for you to quit doing health evangelism in your church for a while. If the problem persists and health evangelism activities are suppressed for a prolonged period of time you might consider transferring your health evangelism activities to another church that will be more receptive.

Under *no* circumstances should you insist on conducting health evangelism in your church if you sense any negativity on the part of the Pastor. I learned this lesson the hard way. I was a full time health evangelist for the local Seventh-day Adventist Church in Towson, Maryland. I was assigned to that church by Elder Bill May, who was president of the Chesapeake Conference at that time. The pastor of the Towson church with whom I thought I was going to work, transferred to the Carolina Conference just the same week I arrived in the church.

The conference assigned a newly baptized, and as not yet ordained pastor, whose background was in journalism, to work with me in the church. This was this pastor's very first church assignment and it was my first church as well. We made attempts to blend our ministry in that little church but it didn't really work out at all. I tried to schedule times for us to study and to pray together but the appointments weren't kept. There were many excuses.

I had an office and medical examination room at the church. We were known as the "Baltimore Healthful Living Center." I am a medical doctor and spent my days working at the church. The pastor spent his days visiting the sick in the hospital. It was role reversal.

We conducted a variety of health evangelism activities on a continuous basis. I planned a speaking part for the pastor in every 5-Day Plan, every cooking school, every weight control program and every exercise program I conducted. The pastor failed to see the evangelistic potential of these health evangelism programs. He just wasn't interested in what I was trying to do in our church. After a couple of months the pastor excused himself from participation in health evangelism and from then on boycotted every program I conducted. He never showed his face again in anything I did in that church.

We had up to 100 non-Adventist participants at every program and the popularity of the Seventh-day Adventist church was growing by leaps and bounds. The church members were excited and were involved with every program we did. I am sorry to report that attendance at prayer meeting dwindled. The pastors influence with his members was falling off.

In my youth and inexperience I went and discussed this with Elder Bill May, the Conference president. He was fully sympathetic with my plight and appreciated the work I was doing in the church. He called the pastor in and read him the riot act. The pastor knew what I had done and was deeply resentful. We never spoke with one another again except on Sabbaths when I attended services.

I didn't know how to remedy this situation until I was instructed by God as to what to do. I was reading the Desire of Ages and had come to the chapter "He Must Increase" that begins on page 178. This chapter describes the conflict that developed between the disciples of John the Baptist and Christ's disciples over the form of the words to be used when conducting a baptismal service. Additionally, John's disciples were concerned with John's decreasing popularity and Christ's ascending popularity.

When John's disciples presented their concerns to John the Baptist his reply was "He must increase, but I must decrease" John 3:30. These were certainly the right words but John did not respond with the correct action and so Jesus did. "Wishing to avoid all occasion for misunderstanding or dissension, He quietly ceased His labors, and withdrew to Galilee." Desire of Ages, 181.

The agenda of the King of the Universe was altered because of a quibble between the disciples of John and Christ. It would be natural for me to think that Christ's response would mirror that of John the Baptist. Christ could well have said. "John must decrease and I must increase." It didn't happen this way. John said the right thing but it didn't solve the problem. The problem was only solved when Jesus and His disciples packed up and moved to Galilee.

When the possibility of conflict arises between you and your pastor and it doesn't appear that harmony can be established, you are advised to do as Christ did when controversy threatened His ministry.

"We also, while loyal to truth, should try to avoid all that may lead to discord and misapprehension. For whenever these arise, they result in the loss of souls.

Whenever circumstances occur that threaten to cause division, we should follow the example of Jesus and of John the Baptist." Desire of Ages, 181.

At this point I reluctantly terminated what I was doing and rapidly transferred my membership to another church about 20 miles away and began health evangelism activities there. The conference terminated it's financial support of my health evangelism activities and I began a very limited practice of medicine to support myself. My work was arranged so I had every evening and every weekend free to conduct health evangelism activities in my new church location.

My leaving Towson was not without the potential for controversy. The head elder who was a strong supporter of health evangelism came to me privately and said. "I know why you are leaving. You and the pastor don't get along. Well, that's too bad. We like what you are doing in our church and we are prepared to FIGHT to keep you here." It was only with considerable effort on my part that we were able to keep the lid on dissension.

Of course, it was natural, and vindictive for me to wish the pastor's efforts to languish once I left the Towson Church. I was humbled when God richly blessed the church once I left. The pastor had record baptisms the next year and the church prospered. I came to rejoice in this.

The point of this long recitation is to emphasize that health evangelism needs to be conducted with the blessing, understanding and cooperation of your local pastor. Don't make the pastor's role in health evangelism too big. Respect that pastors are busy people with many burdens. If the Pastor is against health evangelism, do not do it in his church.

Church Members

Health evangelism activities should largely be conducted by church members. There are many roles for church members in doing medical missionary work. Perhaps the most obvious reason to use church members in conducting health evangelism is their sheer numbers. At this writing the church has more than 12 million members. There are less than 10,000 doctors, less than 30,000 nurses, less than 10,000 dentists and so it goes.

There is an important role for health professionals in conducting health evangelism programs, if they are available in your community. The role of health professionals will be discussed in the next section, but if you just look at the numbers you have, the largest pool of prospective workers is the common ordinary church member who sits in the pew from week to week.

Here is the gold mine of personnel. The local church will always have more members than pastors or health professionals. If you want to have an effective program, plan on filling most of your personnel needs with church members.

Problems with Church Members.

There are certain drawbacks in using church members in conducting health evangelism programs. They should be recognized up front and adjustments made and time taken to develop this resource.

Most church members are not educated in health lines. They have had some basic anatomy and physiology in their schooling but they probably forgot most of what they have learned. This is not a major problem. The church members should learn just about all they need to know about how the body works and what can go wrong during the first program you conduct. Church members will be able to handle most questions and situations in their second or third program.

A bigger problem with some church members is a lack of interest in health evangelism. They are often cold and indifferent as to what is going on in the church. They are too often spiritually weak and are themselves not living up to the light on healthful living that has been shown them in the past.

Some church members are argumentative, hostile and tend to squabble. These types of situations should be resolved before the program begins so a united, cooperative workforce is seen by the public that comes to your health evangelism program. Adequate preparation will resolve most problems.

Many church members are addicted to TV. They would deny it, but if they added up the time devoted to their favorite shows it would consume valuable time that could be spent in doing health evangelism. Many members will decline to help because your schedule will interrupt Monday night football or some other favorite show. Over time, some will be won over to health evangelism but TV can be a barrier to successful medical missionary work.

Some of the most sincere and enthusiastic volunteers will at time be church members who have some limited knowledge of health but have a line of "health products" to sell. They would like to integrate their product line into your health evangelism program. Do not sell vitamins, potions, protein powders, or nutritional supplements at a health evangelism program. Do not allow a church member with a private agenda to push some product in their small group.

And then there are church members who hold some currently popular but scientifically unsound health information which they will want to share with their small group members. Church members should limit the information they discuss in small groups to that which is part of the program. Only qualified health experts should expand on lecture material.

Preparing Church Members

When you first start to conduct health evangelism programs, your personnel will consist of church members who are largely raw recruits who are unskilled. This situation requires a considerable amount of preparation time. Take several weeks to organize and train your church members before you launch into your program.

The time taken in preparation will weed out church members who, after looking at the details of the program you are conducting, will decide that they can't commit to the time it is going to take to do the program. It is sad to see helpers pull out of a program before it even starts but these are the very church members who would be pulling out in the middle of the program leaving you high and dry anyway. It is better to lose helpers before the program begins than to lose them in the midst of a great work.

This was a truth that Gideon learned in Old Testament times, and it is just as true today. Going through a process to remove those who are not dedicated, ill prepared, and half hearted in service will help ensure success

It is best to conduct your training programs on the very same nights of the week that you intend to conduct your health evangelism program. If members can come out to training meetings, they will be able to come out to the program as well. If you conduct your training over a weekend or two, yet your program will be on Tuesday nights, you will find that several who can attend training on the weekend will find that they don't have time to do the program on Tuesday nights for some reason.

The importance of using church members in conducting health evangelism programs is stressed repeatedly in the Spirit of Prophecy writings. Some counsel to consider along these lines is found in the following passages: (emphasis has been added)

> "We have come to a time when *every member* of the church should take hold of medical missionary work. The world is a lazar house filled with victims of both physical and spiritual disease. Everywhere people are perishing for lack of a knowledge of the truths that have been committed to us. The *members of the church* are in need of an awakening, that they may realize their responsibility to impart these truths. Those who have been enlightened by the truth are to be light bearers to the world. To hide our light at this time is to make a terri-

ble mistake. The message to God's people today is: "Arise, shine; for thy light is come, and the glory of the Lord is risen upon thee."" Testimonies for the Church Volume Seven, 62.

There is a sad situation described in the following passage. Church members have had much education and are knowledgeable regarding healthful living. Unfortunately, many, if not most, have not made any significant effort to reform their lives. In doing this they are deliberately choosing evil instead of righteousness. Church members who are not living health reform become agents of Satan and further his cause.

> "We have come to a time when *every member of the church* needs to take hold of medical missionary work. On every hand we see those who have had much light and knowledge and all the advantages that could be given them, deliberately choosing evil in the place of righteousness, mercy, and the love of God. Making no attempt to reform, they are becoming agents of Satan, and are continually growing worse and worse." Manuscript Releases Volume Sixteen, 145.

To live the life of Christ means to do the work he did. This is a work for every member of the church. We are to carry forward the healing and health educational work that He did when he was here.

> "We have come to a time when *every member* of the church should take hold of medical missionary work." "Christ is no longer in this world in person, to go through our cities and towns and villages, healing the sick. He has commissioned us to carry forward the medical missionary work that He began." Testimonies and Experiences Connected with the Loma Linda Sanitarium and College of Medical Evangelists, 7.

What fascinates me most about this next passage is that it specifies who the church member are. Business men, farmers, mechanics, merchants, lawyers and others are singled out here. Each is to advance the cause of Christ by personal effort. Oh, yes, money is mentioned but not as a substitute for personal effort and only after personal effort is mentioned.

> "When men of business, farmers, mechanics, merchants, lawyers, etc., become members of the church, they become servants of Christ; and although their talents may be entirely different, their responsibility to *advance the cause of God by personal effort*, and with their means, is no less than that which rests

upon the minister. The woe which will fall upon the minister if he preach not the gospel, will just as surely fall upon the businessman, if he, with his different talents, will not be a co-worker with Christ in accomplishing the same results. When this is brought home to the individual, some will say, "This is an hard saying;" nevertheless it is true, although continually contradicted by the practice of men who profess to be followers of Christ." Testimonies for the Church Volume Four, 469.

Next we see that the local church is to be organized in such a manner that every member has a work to do. None are to lead an aimless Christian life. All are to be active according to their abilities. This organization is to be accomplished by a thorough organization by the church elders and those who have "leading places" in the church.

"The elders and those who have leading places in the church should give more thought to their plans for conducting the work. They should arrange matters so that *every member* of the church shall have a part to act, that none may lead an aimless life, but that all may accomplish what they can according to their several ability.... It is very essential that such an education should be given to the members of the church that they will become unselfish, devoted, efficient workers for God; and it is only through such a course that the church can be prevented from becoming fruitless and dead.... Let every member of the church become an active worker,—a living stone, emitting light in God's temple." Christian Service, 62.

Church members are able to provide the one-on-one interface that changes lives. Church members can provide the personal labor for souls that is required for success in God's work.

"The Lord desires that His word of grace shall be brought home to every soul. To a great degree this must be accomplished by *personal labor*. This was Christ's method. His work was largely made up of personal interviews. He had a faithful regard for the one-soul audience. Through that one soul the message was often extended to thousands. Christ's Object Lessons, 229.

Church members are to make personal efforts to help those in need. This is accomplished in a health evangelism program by church members providing this personal effort in small groups. Every church member needs to be involved in some type of work. For many this can be through involvement in health evangelism activities.

"Service to God includes personal ministry. By *personal effort* we are to co-operate with Him for the saving of the world. Christ's commission, "Go ye into all the world, and preach the gospel to every creature," is spoken to every one of His followers. (Mark 16:15.) All who are ordained unto the life of Christ are ordained to work for the salvation of their fellow men. Their hearts will throb in unison with the heart of Christ. The same longing for souls that He has felt will be manifest in them. Not all can fill the same place in the work, but *there is a place and a work for all.*" Christ's Object Lessons, 300, 301.

Giving money to the cause of God is not a substitute for personal labor on behalf of those who need our help in overcoming bad habits in their lives.

"Now is our time to labor for the salvation of our fellow men. There are some who think that if they give money to the cause of Christ, this is all they are required to do; the precious time in which they might do *personal service* for Him passes unimproved. But it is the privilege and duty of all who have health and strength to render to God active service. *All are to labor in winning souls to Christ.* Donations of money cannot take the place of this. Christ's Object Lessons, 343.

The work may be small to start with but it should be designed to create a one-on-one contact between church members and the public. This personal influence is powerful. The Holy spirit is present to convict and change minds and lives.

"In every new field, patience and perseverance must be exercised. Be not disheartened at small beginnings. It is often the humblest work that yields the greatest results. The more direct our labor for our fellow-men, the greater good will be accomplished. Personal influence is a power. The minds of those with whom we are closely associated, are impressed through unseen influences. One cannot speak to a multitude and move them as he could if he were brought into closer relationship with them. Jesus left heaven, and came to our world to save souls. You must come close to those for whom you labor, that they may not only hear your voice, but shake your hand, learn your principles, feel your sympathy. Gospel Workers, 340.

While church members do health evangelism, they should do so with kindness and politeness. They should be empathetic. This will result in a hundred fold increase in conversions to the church.

"If we would humble ourselves before God, and be kind and courteous and tenderhearted and pitiful, there would be one hundred conversions to the truth where now there is only one." Testimonies for the Church Volume Nine, 189.

This is an emphatic statement. Church members need to get to work *now*.

> "The world needs *laborers now.* From every direction is heard the Macedonian cry, "Come over and help us." Our success consists in reaching common minds. *Plain, pointed arguments,* standing out as mile-posts, will do more toward convincing people than will a large array of arguments which none but investigating minds will have interest to follow. And if the laborers are pure in heart and life, if they use to the glory of God the talents that he has committed to their keeping, they will have God on their side and heavenly angels to work with their efforts." The Signs of the Times 10-28-1886

Health Professionals

It seems only natural that a health evangelism program would require the services of health professionals wherever possible. While this is ideal, it is not always possible. Health evangelism programs in your church should not be delayed or postponed if you don't have any health professionals among your members.

It is better to utilize the services of health professionals who are members of your own local church than to bring in some specialist from the community or from some long distance. A guest health professional will divert the ownership and authority of the program away from the local church.

A lecture or even just the presence of a health practitioner of any level of education who is a practicing member of your church will be more effective than some highly educated specialist brought in from the outside. It is not so much the quality or quantity of health information that is needed in a health program so much as a clear identification with the local church and involvement of local church members.

Your health evangelism program should be identified with the local church. Outside expertise dilutes this connection. To be more specific, a nurse or a nurse's aide who is a member of your church will be more effective and confirm the local identification of your health evangelism program than a medical doctor or PhD nutritionist you bring in from some distant institution.

The role of the health professional is to provide accurate, scientific, evidence based, factual material relative to health. Health professionals supply information and recommendations about your participant's lifestyle. In a smoking cessation program the information will relate to the health problems associated with smoking and the benefits of quitting. In an exercise program the information will focus on the benefits of exercise. In a nutrition program, foods that are healthful and foods that are unsafe will be reviewed.

If the health professional is well trained and makes a good presentation not only will the participants be educated but the church members who are small group partners will be educated as well. The small groups that meet after the lecture will have a chance to discuss the health information that was presented and to personalize it to their own lives.

The small groups will first review the health information presented by the health professional in the lecture presented a week ago. Partners will determine to what degree implementation of the health information occurred in the lives of the participants since the previous session. Success on the part of the participants is acknowledged and further adherence is encouraged.

The majority of the small group time will be spent in digesting the information just presented in this night's session. The suggestions that were made for behavior change will be discussed by each of the small group members. They will individualize the information to their own experience. You will inquire whether or not the group members are ready to make additional behavior changes based on the health information presented in the lecture.

The small group partners should encourage each member to commit to what they are going to try to do differently in the coming week to carry out the suggestions of the health professional. Health information remains cold and useless unless it is applied to each person's life. The small group is where theory meets commitment to change. Decide what will be practiced in the coming week.

This work cannot be accomplished by the health professional by saying. "Well, that is about it for tonight. Go home and put this into practice." This is what needs to be done but the impact of the lecture is more likely to be put into practice if the topic is discussed and digested in small groups where the group partners will seek for commitments to precise behavior changes from each group member.

The question comes up as to how knowledgeable the small group partners need to be in health topics in order to qualify as small group partners. In my experience, partners don't need health knowledge as much as a compassionate listening ear and a willingness to quietly confront behaviors and ask for a commitment as to what changes each participant is willing to make.

It will be helpful to provide the small group partners with questions they may wish to use to get discussions started and to keep the discussion going. If the small group partners were present and heard the health presentation then they know all they need to know to be group partners for that night.

I always ask the health professional to remain during the small group sessions. They should move around from group to group answering questions that come up to which the small group partners may not know the answer. This takes the pressure off the small group partners to "know it all." Small group partners are also instructed to say, "I don't know but I will try to get an answer by next week" if they don't know the answer to some technical question.

The health professionals you work with don't have to be experts on the topic that is being presented. Any health professional will do. A physical therapist, nurse, dentist, dietician, dental hygienist, health educator or nursing home administrator can present information on the harmful effects of smoking. You don't have to have a board certified oncologist to talk about smoking and lung cancer. You don't need a pulmonary specialist to talk about emphysema.

It may take a health professional who works on the periphery of an issue a bit more time to study up on a given topic but they will do just fine. If the health professional who helps you is a member of your church, it will reinforce in the minds of the participants that your health evangelism program is a local effort made on their behalf. The personal effort of a local group is more appreciated than a polished presentation by some special expert who comes from some distance.

If you don't have any health professionals in your church, then let a layperson give the lecture. You don't have to be a health professional to know that smoking is bad for you and that you ought to eat right and exercise on a regular basis.

If you use a lay person to make the health presentation, it should be acknowledged that he or she is not a trained health professional but keep the apology to a minimum. A layperson who goes to the trouble to learn something about a topic is still more knowledgeable than most of those who are coming for help.

The fact that you are willing to help people with their problems is the most important part of your program. A group of dedicated church members who are willing to come close to individuals who are struggling with problems and to help in any way possible is the fundamental requirement of a successful program.

If you have health professionals in your church, you should invite their participation in every health evangelism program. If you don't have health professionals, you can do health evangelism without them.

One final word of caution. If you are going to conduct a health evangelism program without the services of a health professional the layperson presenting the health information should stick with the basic facts included in the materials of your health program.

Do *not* present any material you download from the Internet unless it is reviewed and approved by a knowledgeable health professional. Do *not* present any material you get from lay magazines especially lay health magazines. There is a lot of true and useful information available on health topics from these sources but it is mixed with so much erroneous material that it is better to stay away from such information unless it can be screened by someone who is skilled in sifting truth from error.

9

Changing Lives

Overview

This is the most important chapter in this book. Behavior change lies at the heart of every self help program. Alcoholics Anonymous helps people quit the use of alcohol. Weight Watchers assists people in losing weight. Smoking cessation clinics help people stop smoking. Nutrition classes are devised to change the way people eat. All health evangelism programs are about behavior changes.

Modern psychological and the therapeutic models have been developed which accurately describe the mental and physical steps people take when they change their behavior. One of these models will be reviewed briefly in this chapter.

It is clear from reading magazines, watching commercials for various products and reading the scientific literature that there are millions who successfully change certain behaviors. The psychological and sociological disciplines have documented the process of behavior change. They have broken the process of change down into various steps which document the processes people go through to improve their lifestyles.

There are limitations with every one of these models. These models are descriptive of behavior changes but their prescriptive value is limited. These behavior change models describe what some people do to change their behavior but these models utterly fail at helping anyone change their behavior. They just don't apply to people who are stuck in a habit or addiction. These models are also unable to motivate people to change.

Here is the problem. Just because some are successful in behavior change doesn't mean that others will be able to follow in their foot steps. Just because you have identified the incremental steps that eventually lead to behavior change in one person doesn't mean that someone else is going to be able to take that same journey. It is partially a matter of motivation. It is partially a matter of capability. Millions want to change things in their life that will result in a healthier way of life but they can't.

Inability to change is fundamentally a spiritual problem that is described in many places in scripture. Perhaps the most famous texts in this regard are the following. "Can the Ethiopian change his skin or the leopard its spots? *Then* may you also do good who are accustomed to do evil" (Jeremiah 13:23).

"For we know that the law is spiritual, but I am carnal, sold under sin. For what I am doing, I do not understand. For what I will to do, that I do not practice; but what I hate, that I do. If, then, I do what I will not to do, I agree with the law that *it is* good. But now, *it is* no longer I who do it, but sin that dwells in me. For I know that in me (that is, in my flesh) nothing good dwells; for to will is present with me, but *how* to perform what is good I do not find. For the good that I will *to do,* I do not do; but the evil I will not *to do,* that I practice. Now if I do what I will not *to do,* it is no longer I who do it, but sin that dwells in me" (Romans 7:14-20).

These texts refer not only to spiritual aspects of our lives but the mental and physical dimensions as well. We all have behaviors that are slowly killing us and we need to change. We all can change some behaviors on our own but every one of us has at least one, and usually multiple behavioral problems that we just can't permanently change no matter how much effort we put forth or how many times we try.

The human will, in and of itself, is not capable of producing permanent change in the life. This applies to the physical and mental dimensions of our life as well as the spiritual. Notice this quotation.

> "But man cannot transform himself by the exercise of his will. He possesses no power by which this change can be effected. The leaven—something wholly from without—must be put into the meal before the desired change can be wrought in it. So the grace of God must be received by the sinner before he can be fitted for the kingdom of glory. All the culture and education which the world can give will fail of making a degraded child of sin a child of heaven. The renewing energy must come from God. The change can be made only by the Holy Spirit. All who would be saved, high or low, rich or poor, must submit to the working of this power. Christ's Object Lessons, 96, 97.

There is a solution for everyone. God has the power to change us. The more times we have failed on our own the more glorious is the deliverance we gain through a relationship with Jesus Christ. This deliverance is what the world needs. Health evangelism programs bring your addictions and bad habits face to face with Christ. Health evangelism programs should do this simply and in a straightforward manner without bringing up more advanced doctrinal issues.

In your health evangelism program do not be hesitant about this. Promise permanent deliverance to everyone who attends your program. This type of deliverance is a miracle. It is our privilege to be the messengers of this good news. The realization of miraculous behavior change will thrill many in your audience and they will testify to the changes that God brought into their lives.

This is a faith-healing service but not in the tradition of the modern faith-healing services we see all around us today. The miracles I see are not a cure for lung cancer but a miraculous deliverance from the tobacco addiction. I don't see cures for cirrhosis of the liver resulting from a life of alcoholism but deliverance from alcoholism through the power of God. I don't see a cure of arthritic knees in the overweight glutton but I do see successful weight loss with God's help. We don't see very many miracles that cure diseases so much as we see miracles resulting in changed behaviors that cause disease.

The church hasn't been very supportive of health evangelism. The church is certain about eternal salvation through Jesus Christ but the church has been decidedly less certain about how Jesus delivers us from harmful behaviors, habits and addictions. Many in the church will deny this, but I ask you to articulate the doctrine of behavior change as it relates to harmful health practices. Sermons aren't preached on this topic. Members are not encouraged to change unhealthy behaviors. There is a considerable difference of opinion among pastors and teachers as to how behavior change is accomplished through a relationship with Jesus.

There is broad agreement that behavior change can occur through a relationship with Jesus but the steps haven't been formalized very well. The details are fuzzy. Most churches and denominations focus on their own unique and distinctive doctrines as these are important for denominational affiliation. Behavior change issues are often postponed until after you accept the doctrines of the church.

Habits and addictions are rather generic problems that equally afflict members of all churches and denominations. I think the fear among many pastors and churches is that focusing on common problems such as obesity, poor nutritional habits, a sedentary lifestyle will result in a label of legalism—a kind of salvation by works. Pastors have told me that church members are already guilt-ridden to begin with. If the church harps on common behavior problems, the guilt would only increase. This could result in negative church growth.

In the following section I will develop the doctrine of how God helps people change behavior. This material is a synthesis of principles from the Holy Bible and the Spirit of Prophecy writings of Ellen G. White. I will also use some concepts on behavior change from a book, *Changing for Good* by J. O. Prochaska, et al. I will utilize some concepts on addiction from the book, *Addiction and Obesity* by G. May, M.D. I will also relate principles from my experience conducting health evangelism programs over the last 30 years.

Awareness of a Problem

There are many people who are simply unaware that they have a behavior that will lead to a loss of health. These people are not necessarily stuck in a bad behavior, they just don't perceive their problem. They have never tried to change their behavior because they don't think they have any bad behaviors.

These people feel safe. They are not afraid of failure. They have no guilt. They don't feel any family or social pressure to change. Some would say that if people aren't aware of something then it really isn't a problem. This is not true. These are a difficult group to reach. Waiting for these people to develop a few symptoms that will wake them up to the reality of their situation is painful for us and risky for them. Too often the first sign of heart disease is sudden death which places a person beyond help.

The longer people wait to change, the more difficult change becomes. The results of a behavior change program are more effective in reducing risk of disease and death when the intervention occurs early in a person's life before permanent damage has been done.

How does one go about motivating people to change who don't know or acknowledge that they even are at risk for anything? These people won't attend a health evangelism program because they don't recognize that there is a problem. What to do? There is something you can do and there is something God can do.

Wake up the unaware by education. A direct appeal might be helpful but you can't push someone into action if they aren't ready to act. Nagging is repetitive and often backfires. At the same time you shouldn't give up your efforts, as apathy on your part may communicate a lack of caring about the problem. Don't be an enabler who helps a problem persist. Don't buy beer, wine, cigarettes, ice-cream, cake or cookies if these are part of the problem.

God is the One who finally wakes us up to our problems and motivates us to change. God works in the life long before we are aware of who He is or our need for His help in our lives. God will bring an awareness of problems in our lives. This may dawn on the mind slowly or suddenly but it will be the drawing, wooing of God that wakes us up to the dangers we face if we persist in health destructive behaviors.

This unconscious drawing of persons to God is described in the following passages:

> "It is true that men sometimes become ashamed of their sinful ways and give up some of their evil habits before they are conscious that they are being drawn to Christ. But whenever they make an effort to reform, from a sincere desire to do right, it is the power of Christ that is drawing them. An influence of which they are unconscious works upon the soul, and the conscience is quickened and the outward life is amended." Mind, Character, and Personality Volume 2, 600.
>
> "Christ is the source of every right impulse. He is the only one that can implant in the heart enmity against sin. Every desire for truth and purity, every conviction of our own sinfulness, is an evidence that His Spirit is moving upon our hearts. Steps to Christ 26.

So where does the motivation for change come from? It comes from God. You should pray that God will wake up those who would benefit from your health evangelism program. You can educate, but unless God wakens the desire for change it won't occur. Be content to leave the unmotivated in the hands of God. God will wake them up in His own good time.

Thinking About Change

Once a person becomes aware of a health problem, he or she begins to think about changing. Thinking about changing behavior represents some progress toward the ultimate goal of healthful living. Those who contemplate change really do want to change. They intend to change someday—but not today. These people are waiting to see if some magic moment will occur that will result in a sudden change in behavior but without much in the way of effort.

Those who want to change worry a lot but don't get around to working on their health problems. They are worried about heart attacks, cancer, obesity, addiction, cirrhosis and on and on but they don't get around to actually doing something about it. These people are worried about cravings, mental anguish, grieving, sadness and loss. Change requires a mental and physical struggle. It takes a high level of motivation to finally get around to doing something about destructive behaviors that lead to disease.

Many who want to change are looking for an easy, foolproof plan that will work for them. A plan is helpful because it organizes the process of change. A plan outlines the steps you take and warns you to lookout for pitfalls of various types. Many will want a plan they can work on in the privacy of their own homes just by themselves. Don't worry about those people. Others will do better in a structured program, in a group setting. Your health evangelism program, conducted in your church will be just what they need.

Preparation for Behavior Change

Many who change will make significant preparation for the process of behavior change. Preparation readies you to take some action and prepares you to handle unexpected challenges. Commitment is the most important element in preparation for change. Commitment is a high level of motivation that fully devotes the will to the process of change. At the point of commitment all ambivalence is lost and courage is high. Certainty of success is in view.

As part of the commitment process, developing and signing a formal contract is often useful. Setting a definite time sets the process of quitting clearly in motion. These concepts can all be incorporated into your health evangelism program.

Going public is often helpful. It is more shameful to fail in front of friends and colleagues if they know about your commitment to change. Going public provides a high level of motivation to not fail. Of course, your health evangelism program is a public program and provides this motivation to your audience.

Action

This is working actively on your problem. Your health evangelism program is all about action. Your program should focus on the process of giving up of old behaviors and working on new behaviors. There are some specific things you can do to help yourself that have a general application to all behavior change. These activities are reviewed here.

Diversions are helpful in getting us to drop old behaviors and in helping us establish new ones. Keep the mind and body busy. Devise activities to occupy the mind with many things that have nothing to do with old behaviors. Focus your energy on new behaviors, projects, and activities. The possibilities are endless.

Exercise is important in helping to change any behavior except exercise addiction. Exercise results in an improved body image. A person experiences increased energy, metabolism and cardiovascular function. Those who exercise have less anxiety and depression and they sleep well. Exercise decreases physical and emotional pain. There are also benefits on body fat and cholesterol levels. Design regular exercise into your health evangelism programs.

Relaxation is an important ingredient in success. Changing behavior is hard emotional and physical work. The battle will often leave one exhausted. There is a need for periods of rest during the struggle. Your prescription should include: early to bed, a quiet work and home environment, body positioning that is comfortable, comfortable clothes, and a letting go, of other concerns that might be a trigger for relapse.

Counter thinking is a mind game. Your mind will suggest dozens of reasons as to why you should return to your old ways. Rehearse positive responses in your mind. Use the logic and authority of your mind to keep you in your new behaviors. Irrational thoughts should be countered by reality.

Prayer is the most important key to success. Prayer will be a new experience for many in your audience. Many who are agnostics, atheists, or nonreligious people will actually try prayer. This is not because they know and believe God but they are in a desperate situation and willing to try almost anything to experience deliverance from their behavioral problem. Of course this is just what God wants. God delights to answer the prayers of all who are struggling. God is willing to surprise someone with success who has never known Him before. What a great way to be introduced to a helping God.

There are two famous texts which have a bearing on behavior change and prayer. A section that follows will deal in greater detail with specifics on the help that God gives to those who ask for help in changing behavior. "Ask, and it will be given to you; seek, and you will find; knock, and it will be opened to you" (Matthew 7:7). "If any of you lacks wisdom, let him ask of God, who gives to all liberally and without reproach, and it will be given to him" (James 1:5).

Mrs. White indicates that when prayer is neglected that temptations creep up on us. Prayer opens up heavens resources which we can use to overcome.

"The darkness of the evil one encloses those who neglect to pray. The whispered temptations of the enemy entice them to sin; and it is all because they do not make use of the privileges that God has given them in the divine appointment of prayer. Why should the sons and daughters of God be reluctant to pray, when prayer is the key in the hand of faith to unlock heaven's storehouse, where are treasured the boundless resources of Omnipotence?" Steps to Christ 94, 95.

When you have prayed for God's help, you need to act on the promise that help will be available to you. You must act as if you have received the help for which you have asked. God's help in overcoming will now be blended with the effort you make and success will be certain.

> "While you pray that you may not be led into temptation, remember that your work does not end with the prayer. You must then answer your own prayer as far as possible, by resisting temptation, and leave that which you cannot do for yourselves for Jesus to do for you. Signs of the Times 11-18-1886.

Assertiveness is helpful. Communicate your thoughts, feelings, wishes and intentions clearly. Positive talk has an effect on your ability to respond. Hearing yourself speak positively helps you to act positively.

It is helpful, as far as possible, *to control the environment* in which you live and work. Avoid people, places or things that might trip you up. This is not a sign of weakness or poor self-control. It is good not to invite temptation but rather avoid it as much as possible. It may not be possible to avoid all tempting situations but remaining steadfast in the face of temptation is easier the more distance and time there is between you and your old habits and addictions.

Avoid cues. Destructive behaviors are usually triggered by certain cues in the environment. Smokers like to light up with a cup of coffee or after a meal. For every habit there are dozens of cues that need to be dealt with. It is good to avoid as many cues as you can. Doing this will be easier if you can identify them in your mind beforehand and if you can practice what you will say or tell yourself if you encounter one of the triggers for your addiction.

It is helpful to leave reminders to yourself in various places. These are *Positive messages* confirming the wisdom of the new behaviors you are modeling. Messages of encouragement to yourself. Reminders strategically placed will go a long way to keep your new behaviors in view and help eclipse the old behaviors you are trying to change.

Rewards are useful. When you give up bad habits, you usually save some money. Reward yourself on a regular basis for the progress you are making. This is important on anniversaries at one week, one month, and one year.

Support from others. Utilize the sympathy and support of family, friends and colleagues as you change. They will be supportive and will lend a listening ear to the struggles you are facing. They will rejoice when you rejoice. These close ones will confirm you in your new behavior and celebrate each victory with you.

God's Special Help with Bad Habits and Addictions

I have already mentioned prayer; but there is much more to learn about God's special help for those who want to overcome. God will help you overcome every bad habit and addiction. God is the answer to life's failures and unfulfilled desires. God wants you to know Him as a helper.

God does not usually save us from the consequences of the diseases we contract from years of indulgence, but God will always help us change our destructive behaviors. You may not know God personally. You may not even believe in God. You may not want to know God, but God wants you to experience Him as a helper in your life. This will be a good test of God's reality for you. If after calling on God you experience success where you had only experienced failure in the past, you will have first hand, personal knowledge that there is a God and that He helps those in need.

Many want unbelievers to come to know Jesus Christ as a redeemer of the "soul" and acknowledge the life, death, and resurrection of Christ as realities before moving on to other issues in the Christian life. This is all well and good but it is rather narrow. In many ways it restricts God's influence and activity in human life.

When Jesus was here on earth working miracles, He opened blind eyes and then the person saw their Savior. Jesus opened the ears of the deaf who then heard the good news of salvation. Healing of disease in Christ's day, in many cases, preceded belief in Christ as Savior. And so today, many who are struggling with destructive habits and addictions can be healed of these deadly behaviors by God as a first step in convincing a person that He is real and is a vital force in his or her life.

God's help is available to all, but God's help will not be dispensed to all. The conditions and circumstances for receiving help from God are very specific yet not unreasonable. It is necessary to become familiar with God's formula for behavior change.

It is important to be positive regarding the outcome of the struggle. Help is at hand. Jesus will be there throughout the struggle. Don't dwell on the negative aspects of behavior change. Fear of consequences discourages but God encourages.

"In working for the *victims of evil habits*, instead of pointing them to the despair and ruin toward which they are hastening, *turn their eyes away to Jesus*. Fix them upon the glories of the heavenly. This will do more for the saving of body and soul than will all the terrors of the grave when kept before the help-less and apparently hopeless." The Ministry of Healing, 62, 63.

I helped conduct a 5-Day Plan to Stop Smoking in Alexandria, Virginia back in the 70's. A participant who was struggling to quit asked about his repeated fail-ures and where and when would he become successful? I was just about to explain God's special help for those who want to quit smoking when a church member frantically waved his hand, wanting to answer the smokers question.

I gave the church member an opportunity to speak and he said, "Lung cancer man, think of lung cancer." The smoker visibly slumped in his chair with a hope-less look on his face. We should inform people of the benefits of behavior change and point the discouraged to God as the One who helps us accomplish what would otherwise be impossible for us to do by ourselves.

God wants us to enjoy the benefits of healthful living. The behavior change God wants us to implement in our lives is not impossible to achieve.

"Our heavenly Father presents before his finite creatures *no impossibilities*; he requires not at their hands that which they cannot perform. He has not set before his church a standard to which they cannot attain; yet he designs that they shall labor earnestly to reach the high standard set before them in the text. He would have them pray that they may be "filled with the fruits of righ-teousness," and then expect this blessing and receive it, and in all things grow up into Christ their living Head." The Signs of the Times, 12-09-1886

Admit You Can't Change on Your Own

Since God is wanting to demonstrate a person's inability to succeed without Him, it is always necessary for those who don't have a relationship with God to come to a realization of their inability to change on their own. If a person is con-fident that he or she can bring about a permanent change for the better in their lives, God doesn't step in to help. A confident person must try again and again until they feel a sense of failure and are convinced of their own inability to change.

This may seem discouraging, but it is a setup for eventual success. If you have failed miserably to change yourself. If you have repeatedly failed to change your-self but you suddenly become successful after calling on God for help you will know that help came from outside yourself. Since success came just after you called on God for help, then God must be real because He reached down and changed you for the better.

This is the point of conversion. It doesn't really matter if you start your walk with God by trusting your lost "soul" to God or your lost physical or mental self to God.

God saves us when we trust Him to save us. Being saved from the sin of smoking is as good a place to start as being saved from the sin of pride. Being saved from a perverted appetite for food, resulting in obesity, is as good a place to start as being saved from some other "spiritual" sin.

A saved person is just a "babe" in Christ. Growth and maturity are necessary to round out the Christian experience. This is known in theological circles as the process of "sanctification." I don't believe any church would be willing to baptize or receive into full fellowship a person whose only experience with God is salvation from smoking but God has saved them and will continue to work with them until they see the "full light" of His salvation.

I want people to know our wonderful God. He loves, He cares, He saves, He changes behavior. I want people to get to know God and they must start somewhere. Where and under what circumstances are people most likely to know God? At some point of disappointment, failure and futility, God will be there to save and change the life.

Yes, baptism and church membership are important in the Christian life; in their own good time. Baptism and church membership are steps in the Christian life that come later on down the line. They do not mark the beginning of the Christian life. Baptism indicates that a person has grown to the point that he or she is ready to join a body of Christian believers.

For unbelievers it is a long walk to the baptismal tank and the right hand of fellowship. That walk must begin at some point in time. Everyone has some type of behavior problem that is keeping them back from personal fulfillment. They have destructive habits, addictions, and strained relationships. Let's introduce these hurting and defeated people to God as the Agent of change in human life.

God will help all defeated people who are willing to call on His name. In the wilderness of Moses time, the poisonous snake bite that resulted in a painful and rapid death was neutralized by a look at the uplifted serpent. So today, the bite of death that comes from drugs, smoking, a sedentary life, alcohol and bad eating habits can all be changed by a look at the uplifted Savior. Jesus changes our behavior. Jesus saves us from our bad behaviors. Jesus saves us. For many, this will begin in a health evangelism program right in your church.

Be Honest with God

God is honest with you and expects you to be honest with Him in return. This is difficult to do. In order to receive God's help with any behavior you want to change, it is necessary for you to be honest with God. God knows you only too well. God only helps those who are honest. So, is there a problem with this? There can be. Think about this implication of honesty.

If God delivers you from cigarette smoking, someone is going to notice your new smoke-free status and ask you if you have quit smoking for good and just how you did it? What is your answer going to be? You may not be a religious person. Up to this point in your life you may have been an atheist or a blasphemer, but now you have experienced some supernatural help. God has just helped you quit smoking. You know you couldn't quit on your own and yet here you are off cigarettes. You asked God to help you not even knowing if there was a God or who God was and yet in a tangible way you have experienced God in your life. Now you are off cigarettes and someone wants to know how you did it. What is your answer going to be? You must be honest in your answer.

It had better be, "I smoked for years and years and tried to quit dozens of times, but without success. I asked God to help me quit and He did it. I am free of this habit due to the specific intervention of God in my life. I am so thankful to God for the deliverance He provided me in this case." That is the truth. God expects you to speak the truth.

In scripture there is the story of a woman who suffered for 12 years with a physical illness. She was healed when she stretched out her hand and anonymously touched the hem of Jesus' garment. This is recorded in Mark 5:25-34. This woman was instantly healed and she would have been satisfied to slip away unnoticed from the crowd. She was content to quietly enjoy God's blessing of healing in the quiet of her own home.

Jesus wanted her to acknowledge that He was the one who healed her. She could have gone home and told the neighbors that she just got over her issue of blood. She could have said that nature healed her in its own good time. She could have bragged on some special diet or herbal supplement she had tried. She could have bragged on some new doctor she had gone to. She really didn't want to publicly acknowledge that it was Jesus who healed her. But when she couldn't hide her healing she spoke up. "But the woman, fearing and trembling, knowing what had happened to her, came and fell down before Him and told Him the whole truth" (Mark 5:33).

When you are healed of some behavioral problem with God's help, you may be fearful and trembling, reluctant to speak for God but God requires you to tell the whole truth. Is this an unfair requirement? Not really. There is a world out there filled with people who need to change and are discouraged due to their many failures. You are to witness to the fact that God changes lives. You are to tell your own story of repeated tries and failures until you achieved success when you eventually asked God for help.

You may believe that there is a God. That alone won't change your life. God is looking for those who need to be changed and who want to be changed. God will change anyone. It doesn't matter if you have a relationship with God at any other level or not. Everyone who eventually comes to know God starts that relationship at some point in time over some problem in life.

Some start their relationship with God in church surrounded by believers and in response to the call of a minister and accompanied by sweet music. We have come to feel that this is the preferred way to meet God. This is all good but it is so limiting.

God will meet you in any place, at any time when you bring a problem to Him that needs to be changed. It doesn't have to be in church although it is especially meaningful if the health evangelism program is conducted in the church because you will be half way home. You may have come to a church just to stop smoking but you met God in a health evangelism program. He is the helper for ALL who are in need of behavior change.

Asking for Help.

The next step in receiving God's help, beyond honesty, is to simply ask God for help. Words need to be spoken. You may have thought about asking God for help. That is not enough. God doesn't respond to a desire on your part. You may have a mental wish that God will help you. God doesn't respond to wishes. Human relationships are formed by an exchange of words. Oh, yes there is body language and a lot is communicated in glances but a formal exchange occurs in words. Often, thoughts and wishes remain vague and nebulous until they are put into words. Putting our desires and requests into words has a way of sharpening and strengthening them. Put your longing for behavior change into words. Speak them aloud. It is often helpful to write them down.

Christians know this process as prayer. This is a word that may scare away those who do not yet have a relationship with God and are not familiar with the process of heavenly communication. It is not necessary to even call this process of talking with God as prayer in your health evangelism program. It is enough to call it talking with God.

God has been leading you for months, years, even your whole life but now is the time to open a return channel. This is done by talking with God. There are no special words that need to be spoken. The conversation should be short and to the point. Here is an example.

"God, I am overweight. I have tried many diets. Some of them worked for a while but never for very long. I look horrible. Obesity is going to ruin my relationship with others. Obesity is going to ruin my health. I want to change. I need to change. I am not able to change permanently by myself. I need help. Please help me lose weight. Oh yes God, I will be honest about this. If You help me lose weight, I will acknowledge that my help came from You. Thank you in advance. Let's get to work."

This is the first of many conversations you will have with God. You will find it necessary to talk with God many times a day. More about this in the section "Keep it up," that follows.

How do you feel now? Perhaps, not a bit different. Only a few suddenly feel victorious. There is no warm glow. There is, usually, no special feeling at all that follows this first talk with God.

If you don't feel anything when you ask God for help, how do you know that God has helped you? When and in what way will you know that God is helping you? What will God's help be like? How long will God's help last? Will God help for one meal, one hour, one day, one week? The answers to these questions are exactly what everyone who is trying to change behavior need to know. The answers to these and other questions follow.

Familiar texts on prayer include the following.

"Ask, and it will be given to you; seek, and you will find; knock, and it will be opened to you. For everyone who asks receives, and he who seeks finds, and to him who knocks it will be opened"(Matthew 7:7,8). "And whatever you ask in My name, that I will do, that the Father may be glorified in the Son. If you ask anything in My name, I will do *it*"(John 14:13,14).

"Now this is the confidence that we have in Him, that if we ask anything according to His will, He hears us" (1 John 5:14).

Prayer is powerful. If prayer can subdue kingdoms, quiet roaring lions and stop fire from consuming, then prayer can help you with your problems and bring about new behaviors.

"The children of God are not left alone and defenseless. Prayer moves the arm of Omnipotence. Prayer has 'subdued kingdoms, wrought righteousness, obtained promises, stopped the mouth of lions, quenched the violence of fire." Christ's Object Lessons, 172.

God is pictured as eagerly leaning forward to catch the plea of one who is struggling to overcome. God has a blessing for us just waiting for us to make our needs known.

> "God is bending from his throne to hear the cry of the oppressed. To every sincere prayer he answers, "Here am I." The prayer that ascends from a broken and contrite heart is never disregarded; it is as sweet music in the ears of our heavenly Father: for he waits to bestow upon us the fulness of his blessing." The Oriental Watchman, 12-01-1909.

God doesn't respond to ceremonious prayers. He wants to hear the frank, desperate, disorganized cry of one facing temptation.

> "There are two kinds of prayer—the prayer of form and the prayer of faith...But the prayer that comes from an earnest heart, when the simple wants of the soul are expressed just as we would ask an earthly friend for a favor, expecting that it would be granted—this is the prayer of faith." My Life Today, 19.

Though God is the Lord of the Universe, He wants us to approach Him as a friend.

> "Prayer is the opening of the heart to God as to a friend. Not that it is necessary in order to make known to God what we are, but in order to enable us to receive Him. Prayer does not bring God down to us, but brings us up to Him." Steps to Christ 93.

You may not know what step to take next. God will guide you to success and equip you to become obedient to the laws of health.

> "Those who decide to do nothing in any line that will displease God, will know, after presenting their case before Him, just what course to pursue. And they will receive not only wisdom, but strength. *Power for obedience*, for service, will be imparted to them, as Christ has promised. Whatever was given to Christ—the "all things" to supply the need of fallen men—was given to Him as the head and representative of humanity. And "*whatsoever we ask, we receive of Him*, because we keep His commandments, and do those things that are pleasing in His sight." 1 John 3:22." The Desire of Ages, 668.

In this struggle to live better, we must overcome the harmful habits we have acquired through life's experiences and even our congenitally acquired tendencies toward bad habits as well. The child of an alcoholic has an addictive personality. This may be overcome through the power of Christ. There are other inherited tendencies that predispose us to harmful behaviors. Many suppose that their natural tendencies are excused or unchangeable because of the laws of nature. This is not true. God has clearly indicated what constitutes healthful behavior. You may have inherited many harmful tendencies but all this can be overcome through the grace of God.

> "It is by the Spirit that the heart is made pure. Through the Spirit the believer becomes a partaker of the divine nature. Christ has given His Spirit as a divine *power to overcome all hereditary and cultivated* tendencies to evil, and to impress His own character upon His church." The Desire of Ages, 671.

There was a lady who attended a 5-Day Plan to Stop Smoking I conducted in Towson, Maryland. I had talked about how God helps smokers quit. After the program I was talking with this lady in the parking lot of the church. She lit up a cigarette and was smoking. She said, "I have been asking God to help me stop smoking for the past 20 years and He hasn't done it."

This lady and I had a little discussion about what she expected God to do in helping her to quit. I asked whether she expected God to make her lighter so it wouldn't light? Was she expecting matches to fizzle and go out before she could light up? Was she expecting God to jam all the cigarette machines when she tried to buy cigarettes? Did she expect God to work on the mind of the checkout clerk at the local store when she tried to buy cigarettes, so the checkout person would refuse to sell her any cigarettes because God was trying to get her to quit?

She was repeatedly asking God to help her quit smoking but without her having to do anything. She was expecting God to force her to stop smoking in response to her prayer. Prayer doesn't work that way. God doesn't work that way. This lady needed to act on her request to God. She needed to act like she was a nonsmoker. This is discussed next.

Application

Immediately after asking God for help comes the time for action on your part. You should have a plan of action based on the suggestions made in the previous section on "Action." For the obese person, that plan will include a diet and some eating behavior changes. For the smoker it is time to throw away the cigarettes, lighters and ash trays. For the sedentary person it is initiating a regular program of exercise. For the alcoholic it may be attending an Alcoholics Anonymous meeting. For those with a bad temper it may be an anger management program. For those attending your health evangelism program you will be providing the plan of action a person needs to follow.

Having to work at behavior change may seem too familiar to you. You have done this before. You know what a tremendous effort and strain it is. For you, diet or exercise programs, and in fact all programs you have ever tried have been frustrating and did not produce lasting success.

What is going to be the difference between this program any the many others you have tried in the past? The difference is that you have asked God to help you. God does not dispense with your effort or cooperation when He provides help for you to overcome. God works with your efforts. God helps you work the plan you intend to follow. Have a plan and put it to work. God is right there with you to make it successful this time.

So, if you have a plan and are working it, do you now have a brighter vision of success? Are you brimming with confidence? Do you know that this plan is going to work for you this time? Probably not. So when will you know that God has been helping you? When and in what ways will you experience God's help?

The simple answer is, "Just when you need it, God's help will be there." God's presence and influence acting in the human life is often not felt at the time the plea for help is made. But, God's action in your behalf will show up when you need it. You will experience God's special help on your behalf. God will help you but only if you are taking some action in your own behalf.

There are several illustrations of this point in scripture. These are examples of where God manifested miraculous power on behalf of a person but a cooperative effort was required on the part of the person or persons at hand at the time the miracle was performed.

The raising of Lazarus is a prime example. This is recorded in John 11. The story is a familiar one to many. Raising Lazarus to life, four days after he died, was Christ's greatest miracle. As Jesus stood at the tomb He instructed that the stone be rolled away. This command to remove the stone seems strange to me.

It takes less divine power to move a stone than it does to raise a person from the dead. It would have added significant drama to the scene if the stone had mysteriously moved all by itself or been shattered with a bolt of lightening.

The point is this, in every miracle God performs, there is a part for us to play. God will not do for us what we can do for ourselves. Jesus required someone to roll away the stone from the opening of the tomb. Martha objected to removing the stone. If there had been a lot of sympathy for Martha's point of view and a general outcry had developed for the stone to stay in place; I don't believe that Lazarus would have been raised from the dead.

I repeat, there is a part for us to do in every miracle. Now, I don't think the men who rolled away the stone went home that evening and boasted to their family how they and Jesus had raised Lazarus from the dead. Everyone knows that rolling stones around in the graveyard never brought anyone to life. Yet if the stone didn't get rolled away Lazarus wouldn't have been raised.

The part we play in any miracle is absolutely necessary for the miracle to happen but it has absolutely nothing to do with the power it takes to perform the miracle. All the power comes from God but, our cooperation is necessary. Our efforts are acts of faith moving or even just leaning in the direction we want to go, but God supplies all the ability.

Another example is when Jesus turned water into wine at the wedding feast in Cana. This is recorded in John 2. Jesus required those household servants to fill the water jars with water and then dip it out and serve it. The water was then suddenly turned into wine.

If the servants had objected and refused to fill the jars with water there wouldn't have been any wine. When those servants went home that night, they certainly recounted to their families what a great miracle Jesus had performed, but I doubt they took any credit for the miracle because you can fill jars with water all your life, and it will never turn to wine unless there is a miracle from God.

I am repeatedly making the point that it is necessary for people to participate in the performance of a miracle. If we don't do our part, God doesn't do His part. Our part is essential but ineffectual. God does it all but waits for us to cooperate with him.

Let me give you a third example to make this point perfectly clear. When the children of Israel crossed the Jordan river, they all marched forward even though the river was at flood stage. This is recorded in Joshua 3. There was no bridge and no boats. They lined up and marched forward. They could have waited until they saw a dry river bed before they walked through the Jordan. Looking out of their tents each day they could have said, "Oh, well, the water looks pretty high today—may be tomorrow will be a better day." If they had refused to march forward there never would have been a miracle.

The children of Israel all lined up and headed in the direction they wanted to go. When the feet of the priests touched the flood waters, the Jordan was held back and they all crossed over on dry ground. A miracle happened. The people marched forward indicating a willingness to do what God requested. God provided the miracle. Again we see the cooperation between the human and the Divine. Man acted as though God was going to do something, and He did. God requires us to act and then He provides ALL the power to accomplish the act.

Mrs. White indicates that cooperation between the human and the Divine is necessary in order to form a correct character. It is clear that we must make serious efforts but that our own efforts are not sufficient to accomplish anything. We are still wholly dependent on God for Success.

> "The work of gaining salvation is one of copartnership, a joint operation. There is to be co-operation between God and the repentant sinner. This is necessary for the formation of right principles in the character. Man is to make earnest efforts to overcome that which hinders him from attaining to perfection. But he is wholly dependent upon God for success. Human effort of itself is not sufficient. Without the aid of divine power it avails nothing. God works and man works. Resistance of temptation must come from man, who must draw his power from God. On the one side there is infinite wisdom, compassion, and power; on the other, weakness, sinfulness, absolute helplessness." The Acts of the Apostles, 482

Human effort is worthless unless energized by divine power. Divine help is unavailable unless there is human effort.

> "Human effort avails nothing without divine power; and without human endeavor, divine effort is with many of no avail. To make God's grace our own, we must act our part. His grace is given to work in us to will and to do, but never as a substitute for our effort.... Those who walk in the path of obedience will encounter many hindrances. Strong, subtle influences may bind them to the world; but the Lord is able to render futile every agency that works for the defeat of His chosen ones; in His strength they may overcome every temptation, conquer every difficulty." God's Amazing Grace, 253

There are certain actions essential for success which we must do. We can speak the right words and can take certain actions toward the goal we want to accomplish. These actions themselves are gifts which we have already received from God. The use of these talents and skills help us move in the direction we want to go. God will not duplicate that which He has already enabled us to do.

> "The Lord does not propose to perform for us either the willing or the doing. This is our proper work. As soon as we earnestly enter upon the work, God's grace is given to work in us to will and to do, but never as a substitute for our

effort. Our souls are to be aroused to cooperate. The Holy Spirit works the human agent, to work out our own salvation. This is the practical lesson the Holy Spirit is striving to teach us. "For it is God which worketh in you both to will and to do of His good pleasure." Testimonies to Ministers and Gospel Workers, p. 240

In all our efforts to overcome bad habits we must constantly be aware that we are weak and success at this moment does not guarantee our success in the next hour or tomorrow. We need God's constant help but must never let down our guard or relax our own efforts to succeed.

"In order to receive God's help, man must realize his weakness and deficiency; he must apply his own mind to the great change to be wrought in himself; he must be aroused to earnest and persevering prayer and effort. Wrong habits and customs must be shaken off; and it is only by determined endeavor to correct these errors and to conform to right principles that the victory can be gained. Patriarchs and Prophets p. 248

As we make constant earnest struggles, we should be looking to and contemplating the goodness of God and how it is His strength that enables us to be successful.

"Let every one who desires to be a partaker of the divine nature appreciate the fact that he must escape the corruption that is in the world through lust. There must be a constant, earnest struggling of the soul against the evil imaginings of the mind. There must be a steadfast resistance of temptation to sin in thought or act. The soul must be kept from every stain, through faith in Him who is able to keep you from falling. We should meditate upon the Scriptures, thinking soberly and candidly upon the things that pertain to our eternal salvation. The infinite mercy and love of Jesus, the sacrifice made in our behalf, call for most serious and solemn reflection. We should dwell upon the character of our dear Redeemer and Intercessor. We should seek to comprehend the meaning of the plan of salvation. We should meditate upon the mission of Him who came to save His people from their sins. By constantly contemplating heavenly themes, our faith and love will grow stronger. Our prayers will be more and more acceptable to God, because they will be more and more mixed with faith and love. They will be more intelligent and fervent." Sons and Daughters of God, 109.

There are stern battles with self that need to be fought. We need to examine our progress regularly. God gives us the talents and the powers of mind that we can use in developing our habit-free character.

"But Christ has given us no assurance that to attain perfection of character is an easy matter. A noble, all-round character is not inherited. It does not come to us by accident. A noble character is earned by individual effort through the merits and grace of Christ. God gives the talents, the powers of the mind; we form the character. It is formed by hard, stern battles with self. Conflict after conflict must be waged against hereditary tendencies. We shall have to criticize ourselves closely, and allow not one unfavorable trait to remain uncorrected. Christ's Object Lessons, 331.

It is amazing to me that with God's help that even hereditary traits can be corrected. Think of the health problems and harmful practices for which a congenital component has been identified. All this can be changed.

"Through the Spirit the believer becomes a partaker of the divine nature. Christ has given His Spirit as a divine power to overcome all hereditary and cultivated tendencies to evil, and to impress His own character upon His church." The Desire of Ages, 671

When we have done all that we can, God will do all that we can't.

"Some reason that the Lord will by his Spirit qualify a man to speak as he would have him; but the Lord does not propose to do the work which he has given man to do. He has given us reasoning powers, and opportunities to educate the mind and manners. And after we have done all we can for ourselves, making the best use of the advantages within our reach, then we may look to God with earnest prayer to do by his Spirit that which we cannot do for ourselves, and we shall ever find in our Saviour power and efficiency. Gospel Workers, 148.

Constant watchfulness, persevering effort, severe discipline and tough conflict will be our lot, but as we depend on God we can right the deformity of our characters. There is a lifetime of struggle, but with God's help the outcome is certain.

"It will cost us an effort to secure eternal life. It is only by long and persevering effort, sore discipline, and stern conflict, that we shall be overcomers. But if we patiently and determinedly, in the name of the Conqueror who overcame in our behalf in the wilderness of temptation, overcome as he overcame, we shall have the eternal reward. Our efforts, our self-denial, our perseverance, must be proportionate to the infinitive value of the object of which we are in pursuit.... Wrongs cannot be righted, nor reformations in character made, by a few feeble, intermittent efforts. Sanctification is not a work of a day or a year, but of a lifetime. Without continual efforts and constant activity, there can be no advancement in the divine life, no attainment of the victor's crown.... You have need of constant watchfulness, lest Satan beguile you through his subtlety, corrupt your minds, and lead you into inconsistencies and gross darkness. Your watchfulness should be characterized by a spirit of humble dependence upon God. It should not be carried on with a proud, self-reliant spirit, but with a deep sense of your personal weakness, and a childlike trust in the promises of God." Gospel Workers, 205.

Living a healthful live is not an option. Once we know what should be done we need to act.

"The time of ignorance God winked at, but as fast as light shines upon us, He requires us to change our health-destroying habits, and place ourselves in a right relation to physical laws." Counsels on Diet and Foods, 19.

There is a need for struggle and perseverance. "Those who, after seeing their mistakes, have courage to change their habits will find that the reformatory process requires a struggle and much perseverance;" Counsels on Diet and Foods, 24.

Temptation

Temptation shows up in many ways depending on what you are trying to overcome. For the smoker who is trying to quit there is a craving for cigarettes. For the alcoholic it is a craving for the numbing nothingness that alcohol brings to the battered brain. For the sedentary it is the urge to stay in bed and not hit the jogging trail. For the obese it is the urge to snack or perhaps temptations for second helpings of a particularly delicious dish. For those with anger issues it is an urge to yell at a stupid employee, family member or careless driver on the road. For the sex addict it is the drawing of the eyes to pornography on the Internet or in magazines. To the lazy it is a line up of entertaining TV programs for the evening. For the spiritually indolent it may be missing church or Sabbath School or prayer meeting or omission of daily devotions.

These are all temptations. Temptations result in the downfall of many. Temptations are the barrier between you and success. Temptations are often resisted for a few hours, days, weeks or even years but then at some point of weakness you give in and experience failure once again. Here is where you need God's help in overcoming.

What does God do about temptations? Well, if you didn't ask God for help, God isn't going to do anything about your temptations. If you did ask God for help, you are about to succeed where you only experienced failure before. Does God help with every temptation? Does God help with big temptations but leave the small ones up to you? You are about to find out.

Temptations come in various sizes and intensities. There are small brief temptations that come when you are busy. Something crosses your mind but because you are so busy you barely give the temptation a passing thought. I believe these kinds of temptation will be with us all of our lives. God does not prevent us from being tempted. In fact, God allows us to be tempted. Satan tempts us to bring out the worst in us, but God allows temptation to bring out the best in us.

As long as we are in this world we will be subject to temptation. Being a child of God does not exempt us from temptation, but being a child of God puts resources at our disposal we can use to resist temptation. When we ask God for help in overcoming some destructive behavior, we can expect frequent and intense temptations that we can successfully meet and overcome with God's help.

Fortunately, over time, temptations about a specific problem tend to become less intense and less frequent, but even after several months or years of successful living, temptations can return in strength. This is not a sign that God has abandoned us. It is a sign that Satan hasn't given up on us yet and is determined to break us down in one way or another. The reason temptations come less and less frequently with time is that when Satan finds he is unable to overcome us in one area he shifts his efforts to some other area of weakness in our life and starts a blizzard of temptations regarding some other problem in the hopes of breaking us down one way or another.

For instance, when a person stops smoking, in addition to temptations to return to smoking, there is a tendency on the part of many to want to eat more. Food tastes better when you aren't smoking. The hand-to-mouth motions of eating are similar to the actions of smoking. I have seen people put on 30 or 40 pounds after quitting smoking. It is good to stop smoking but it is bad to become a glutton as a consequence. Here, one bad habit replaced another. This is how Satan works. Temptations in one area may decrease only to be replaced by a whole new set of temptations in some other area of life.

So, where and when does God help us when we are fighting with temptation? God doesn't very often remove a temptation altogether. God may not reduce the frequency of temptation. God may not reduce the intensity of temptation. But God does keep us from yielding to temptation and falling back into our old ways.

In some cases God will totally eliminate all temptation about a certain problem. In one of my stop smoking clinics I had a man who quit smoking with God's help. I saw him several months later and he said that God totally eliminated the desire for tobacco from him. He didn't have a single craving or desire for tobacco at any time since he committed the problem to God. I believe this man. It was a wonderful deliverance that God performed in his life. God can do this for anyone and God may do this for you. I warn you however, this type of deliverance is unusual.

God usually lets a person be tempted and get pretty close to failure before stepping in. There is a certain intensity of temptation where you have always failed before. You know where this point is, and you know when you are getting close to it. God can and may intervene in your temptation at any point before the point of failure. But surely, God will not let you fail if you have committed this problem to Him. You will see what God will do in your life.

If God doesn't seem to be doing much about your temptation, do not despair. God will not let you fail. There is a point where God *always* steps in and gives you success. God will *always* intervene and turn back your temptation; if not early in the temptation, at least God will step in with relief just before you reach the point of failure. You may think you have reached the breaking point but here is where God will certainly bring you success.

God will not let you fail. You asked God for help and here it is. Just when you feel you have reached the point of failure, God will enable you to say NO to your temptation. At just the point where you have always failed before you will now always have success. This is where God's help shows up for sure. Instead of experiencing repeated failures as you did in the past you will now experience victory.

Why does God wait until the point of failure before He steps in? There are several reasons why God may allow this to be your experience. All these reasons for temptation need to be understood.

One reason for intense temptations has to do with your honesty and sincerity. God is creating a record of your life. Your words, actions and motives are all recorded. For the committed Christian, words and actions match up. For many, unfortunately, words are often braver than deeds.

Words are cheap. You may ask for God's help, but Satan is trying to prevent you from receiving God's help. Satan may be saying to God, "Don't interrupt this temptation just yet. She is not honest. She is not sincere. Just let the temptation develop a little bit more and she will give in as usual. This temptation is mild. She has successfully resisted similar temptations in the past and doesn't really need Your help just yet. Watch her for just a few seconds more because she is just about to give in. She may say that she wants Your help, but those are just words. Watch and see what she does."

God wants to demonstrate your honesty and sincerity before the universe before He steps in to help. For this reason your temptations may be strong on occasion. You may become very uncomfortable. It is good to keep in mind that every effort you make in your own behalf is a measure of your honesty and sincerity. To be sure, every effort you make in your own behalf is totally inadequate to keep you from falling back into bad behaviors and your best effort has never been able to deliver you in the past, but it is a measure of the intensity of your desire to receive God's help. God honors that and will not let you fail.

Here are a few texts that bear out the truth of these words. "No temptation has overtaken you except such as is common to man; but God *is* faithful, who will not allow you to be tempted beyond what you are able, but with the temptation will also make the way of escape, that you may be able to bear *it*" (1 Corinthians 10:13).

In the Lord's Prayer we are admonished to pray about temptations and to ask for deliverance from them. "And do not lead us into temptation, But deliver us from the evil one. For Yours is the kingdom and the power and the glory forever. Amen" (Matthew 6:13).

Jesus reminded his disciples that by prayer they would be able to avoid or overcome temptation. "Watch and pray, lest you enter into temptation. The spirit indeed *is* willing, but the flesh *is* weak" (Matthew 26:41).

Another safeguard against temptation is contained in the parable of the sower in Luke 8. This describes those who have heard the good news but who are overcome by temptation. These start out well, but because they remain superficial in their experience and don't advance in their relationship with God, they are unprepared for severe temptations. "But the ones on the rock *are those* who, when they hear, receive the word with joy; and these have no root, who believe for a while and in time of temptation fall away" (Luke 8:13).

Temptations have a purpose. If we maintain our hold on God and with His help endure temptations, we will be approved by God and will receive the crown of life. This may be the experience of those who learn to trust God at a health evangelism program: "Blessed *is* the man who endures temptation; for when he has been approved, he will receive the crown of life which the Lord has promised to those who love Him" (James 1:12).

It is my reasoning that the next text applies to those who are trying to overcome temptation. Some would argue that a secular person doesn't have the opportunity or right to apply this text to his or her life because they have not been born of God. My point is that being born of God occurs at the point where you avail yourself of God's help. Being born of God is associated with altar calls at evangelistic meetings in response to a broad understanding of distinctive doctrines, but it must be applied as well to the person who, for the first time, claims God's special help for a problem area in the life. "For whatever is born of God overcomes the world. And this is the victory that has overcome the world—our faith" (1 John 5:4).

In referring to the temptation of Peter, Mrs. White indicates that in the Christian life the Lord does not save us from trial but does save us from defeat.

> "It was necessary for Peter to learn his own defects of character, and his need of the power and grace of Christ. The Lord could not save him from trial but He could have saved him from defeat…he would have received divine help so that Satan could not have gained the victory." Christ's Object Lessons, 155.

Once we have entered the struggle to overcome a bad habit there will be many situations that will come up to divert us from the problem we are trying to overcome. We will be successful as we keep our mind on Christ.

> "You have Satan to contend with, and he will seek by every possible device to attract your mind from Christ. But we must meet all obstacles placed in our way, and overcome them one at a time. If we overcome the first difficulty, we shall be stronger to meet the next, and at every effort will become better able to make advancement. By looking to Jesus, we may be over comers. It is by fastening our eyes on the difficulties and shrinking from earnest battle for the right, that we become weak and faithless. The Youth's Instructor, 01-05-1893.

Many who avail themselves of God's help will eventually fail to overcome their bad habits. This is not God's fault or the fault of your health evangelism program.

> "Those who work for the fallen will be disappointed in many who give promise of reform. Many will make but a superficial change in their habits and practices. They are moved by impulse, and for a time may seem to have reformed; but there is no real change of heart. They cherish the same self-love, have the same hungering for foolish pleasures, the same desire for self-indulgence. They have not a knowledge of the work of character building, and they cannot be relied upon as men of principle. They have debased their mental and spiritual powers by the gratification of appetite and passion, and this makes them weak. They are fickle and changeable. Their impulses tend

toward sensuality. These persons are often a source of danger to others. Being looked upon as reformed men and women, they are trusted with responsibilities and are placed where their influence corrupts the innocent." The Ministry of Healing, p. 177.

We can overcome some temptations by ourselves on certain occasions but we can't have long term success without God's help. God expects us to recognize our weakness yet make determined efforts to correct our faults and errors.

"In order to receive God's help, man must realize his weakness and deficiency; he must apply his own mind to the great change to be wrought in himself; he must be aroused to earnest and persevering prayer and effort. Wrong habits and customs must be shaken off; and it is only by determined endeavor to correct these errors and to conform to right principles that the victory can be gained. Many never attain to the position that they might occupy, because they wait for God to do for them that which He has given them power to do for themselves. All who are fitted for usefulness must be trained by the severest mental and moral discipline, and God will assist them by uniting divine power with human effort." Patriarchs and Prophets, 248.

Satan may tempt us, but Satan can't make us give in to temptation. Christ repulsed temptation and will give us strength to meet all temptations as well.

"Satan assailed Christ with his fiercest and most subtle temptations, but he was repulsed in every conflict. Those battles were fought in our behalf; those victories make it possible for us to conquer. Christ will give strength to all who seek it. No man without his own consent can be overcome by Satan. The tempter has no power to control the will or to force the soul to sin. He may distress, but he cannot contaminate. He can cause agony, but not defilement. The fact that Christ has conquered should inspire His followers with courage to fight manfully the battle against sin and Satan. The Great Controversy, 510.

Keeping it up

Success comes a day at a time. Success today may be followed by failure tomorrow but this need not be. Success today is proof that we can be successful tomorrow as well. The formula that worked today will also work tomorrow. At times we fail because we fail to maintain our connection with God. We start out well, but don't keep it up.

I had a lady in my office practice who had successfully lost 40 pounds with God's help. She was so happy. She had never lost more than 5 pounds on any diet in the past. She was praying to God every day and God was giving her success.

One day, this lady came into my office and was a bit concerned. She said, "If I don't pray to God at breakfast, I overeat at breakfast. If I don't pray at noon, I over eat at lunch time. If I don't pray at dinner time, I overeat in the evening. If I don't pray to God all the time this just doesn't work!" She was upset and brought her fist down forcefully on my desk.

We had a long discussion about the nature of God's help. God is willing to help us as long as we maintain a relationship with Him. If we lose our contact with God we will rather immediately revert to our old behaviors. God is desiring a long term relationship with us. As long as we maintain our connection with Him, He is actively working on our behalf. I explained that God admonishes us to "pray without ceasing." "Rejoice always, pray without ceasing, in everything give thanks; for this is the will of God in Christ Jesus for you"(1 Thessalonians 5:16-18).

This lady immediately saw the significance of what I was saying. She realized that she was complaining about having to maintain a continuous connection with God. She brightened and said she would never again complain about having to maintain contact with God. I am pleased to report that she kept her weight off until the time of her death some time later.

It is wearisome at times to keep focused on your problem and to constantly be in prayer to God. It is easy to be diverted from our important goals. With time however, we become accustomed to being in God's presence and learn to depend on Him at all times for all things. Jesus admonishes us to take His yolk upon us. "Take My yoke upon you and learn from Me, for I am gentle and lowly in heart, and you will find rest for your souls" (Matthew 11:29).

In order for us to always succeed we must continue to keep the Lord always before us.

"The reason why so many are left to themselves in places of temptation is that they do not set the Lord always before them. When we permit our communion with God to be broken, our defense is departed from us. Not all your good purposes and good intentions will enable you to withstand evil. You must be men and women of prayer. Your petitions must not be faint, occasional, and fitful, but earnest, persevering, and constant. It is not always necessary to bow upon your knees in order to pray. Cultivate the habit of talking with the Saviour when you are alone, when you are walking, and when you are busy with your daily labor. Let the heart be continually uplifted in silent petition for help, for light, for strength, for knowledge. Let every breath be a prayer. The Ministry of Healing, 510,511.

We should plan on obtaining a new victory every day.

"God is our strength. We must look to Him for wisdom and guidance, and keeping in view His glory, the good of the church, and the salvation of our own souls, we must overcome our besetting sins. We should individually seek to obtain new victory every day. We must learn to stand alone and depend wholly upon God. The sooner we learn this the better. Let each one find out where he fails, and then faithfully watch that his sins do not overcome him, but that he gets the victory over them. Then can we have confidence toward God, and great trouble will be saved the church." Early Writings of Ellen G. White 105.

Keeping up with successful living results from abiding in Christ and thorough continual communication with Him.

"This union with Christ, once formed, must be maintained. Christ said, "Abide in Me, and I in you. As the branch cannot bear fruit of itself, except it abide in the vine; no more can ye, except ye abide in Me." This is no casual touch, no off-and-on connection. The branch becomes a part of the living vine. The communication of life, strength, and fruitfulness from the root to the branches is unobstructed and constant. Separated from the vine, the branch cannot live. No more, said Jesus, can you live apart from Me. The life you have received from Me can be preserved only by *continual communion*. Without Me you *cannot overcome one sin, or resist one temptation*. The Desire of Ages, 676.

If we have learned to abide in Christ, we will identify new problems in our lives that need to be corrected, and we can overcome each one through the strength that Christ provides. This will result in a string of uninterrupted victories.

"Christ rejoiced that He could do more for His followers than they could ask or think. He spoke with assurance, knowing that an almighty decree had been given before the world was made. He knew that truth, armed with the omnipotence of the Holy Spirit, would conquer in the contest with evil; and that the bloodstained banner would wave triumphantly over His followers. He knew that the life of His trusting disciples would be like His, a series of uninterrupted victories, not seen to be such here, but recognized as such in the great hereafter. The Desire of Ages, 679.

Those situations which seem sure to trip us up will disappear as we make a consistent effort to do the will of God.

> "Those who would walk in the path of obedience to God's commandments will encounter many hindrances. There are strong and subtle influences that bind them to the ways of the world; but the power of the Lord can break these chains. He will remove these obstacles from before the feet of his faithful, humble children, or give them strength and courage to conquer every difficulty, if they earnestly beseech his help. *All hindrances will vanish before an earnest desire and persistent effort to do the will of God.* Light from Heaven will illuminate the pathway of those who, no matter what trials and perplexities they may encounter, go forward in the way of obedience, looking to Jesus for help and guidance. The Signs of the Times, 07-22-1886

There was another lady who was visiting with me after a Smoking Cessation Clinic. She was smoking in the parking lot just before she left for the evening. She had heard what I had said about how God helped smokers quit. She remarked to me, "I quit smoking with God's help."

I was surprised because she was smoking as she told me this. I asked her, "What happened?" She said that after about six months she decided she could stay off cigarettes all by herself. She felt she didn't need God's help with smoking anymore. Well, obviously she had failed, because she was smoking as she was talking with me.

I next asked her, "What do you plan to do about your smoking?" Her response was, "I will just keep trying." Notice the "I." She was determined to quit on her own and was not meeting with any success. It is my belief that she will never be able to quit smoking on her own. She needs to find God again. She needs to start working with God once again. She knows just where she left Him and she knows exactly what help is available.

Thankfulness

Another key to long-lasting success is being thankful for the success you have experienced. If you go an hour without smoking, that represents success and you should thank God for what He has done for you. If you go a whole day without smoking, it is time to thank God for what He is doing for you.

If you have asked God to help you overcome an addiction or habit and you now have had the problem under control for a few days, how do you know that God is in fact helping you? You may not feel very different from what you did before you changed. The first level of proof that God is helping you is that you aren't doing what you used to do. You are living a successful life.

At this point some people want to think that they are actually the ones that are responsible for their own success. This is a serious mistake that leads to failure. The best way to avoid this mistake is to be thankful to God for all success.

After an hour without a cigarette, thank God for success. After a day without snacking or overeating, thank God for success. After a day without drugs, pornography, or alcohol, thank God for success. The more we thank God for what He is doing for us the more convinced we will be that it is He who is helping us and not we ourselves.

Scripture advises us to be thankful for what God has accomplished for us. "But God be thanked that *though* you were slaves of sin, yet you obeyed from the heart that form of doctrine to which you were delivered. And having been set free from sin, you became slaves of righteousness" (Romans 6:17,18). "But thanks *be* to God, who gives us the victory through our Lord Jesus Christ. Therefore, my beloved brethren, be steadfast, immovable, always abounding in the work of the Lord, knowing that your labor is not in vain in the Lord" (1 Corinthians 15:57, 58). "Now thanks *be* to God who always leads us in triumph in Christ, and through us diffuses the fragrance of His knowledge in every place. For we are to God the fragrance of Christ among those who are being saved and among those who are perishing" (2 Corinthians 2:14,15). "Be anxious for nothing, but in everything by prayer and supplication, with thanksgiving, let your requests be made known to God; and the peace of God, which surpasses all understanding, will guard your hearts and minds through Christ Jesus" (Philippians 4:6, 7). "And *whatever* you do in word or deed, *do* all in the name of the Lord Jesus, giving thanks to God the Father through Him" (Colossians 3:17). "Rejoice always, pray without ceasing, in everything give thanks; for this is the will of God in Christ Jesus for you" (1 Thessalonians 5:16-18).

There are many reminders to be thankful to God in the Spirit of Prophecy writings. "Thank God with soul and voice; and say, "I thank God that I am alive; I thank God for my reason; I thank God for physical strength that I may speak and act under his supervision." Advent Review and Sabbath Herald, 11-14-1893

We should thank God that we are not left alone in the struggle to change our behavior.

"To every Christian comes the word that was addressed to Peter, "Satan hath desired to have you, that he may sift you as wheat: but I have prayed for thee, that thy faith fail not." Luke 22:31. *Thank God we are not left alone.* This is our safety. Satan can never touch with eternal disaster one whom Christ has prepared for temptation by His previous intercession; for grace is provided in Christ for every soul, and a way of escape has been made, so that no one need fall under the power of the enemy. Our High Calling, 311.

Summary

As I bring this chapter to a close, I want to make sure you understand what we have said here. The points are these.

1. Some people can change some of their behavioral problems by themselves. But someday they will find a problem that they won't be able to change without God's help.

2. God helps people change their behavior. This introduction to God as the agent of change in human life can occur in a health evangelism program that is otherwise free of distinctive doctrines.

3. God requires persons to be honest and truthful.

4. God requires people to ask for help.

5. God requires people to make efforts to change their behavior. God's grace provides success as we make efforts to help ourselves. A person who does this is converted and has tasted God's salvation.

6. God requires people to maintain their contact with Him. Long term results come from a long term relationship with God.

7. Thankfulness is the way you attribute the success you enjoy to God.

10

A Biblical Model of Health Evangelism

There is a story in the Old Testament of the Bible that perfectly illustrates all of the various elements of health evangelism as outlined in this book. The use of Old Testament stories to learn how to work today is justified by Paul in the following texts.

"Now all these things happened to them as examples, and they were written for our admonition, upon whom the ends of the ages have come" (1 Corinthians 10:11).

"For whatever things were written before were written for our learning, that we through the patience and comfort of the Scriptures might have hope" (Romans 15:4).

The following story tells us how to do health evangelism and is found in 2 Kings 4:1-7. I have spiritualized the various elements in this story. You will see how God wants us to work for others in the local church. I am going to analyze this passage verse by verse and word by word.

2 Kings 4:1

"A certain woman of the wives of the sons of the prophets cried out to Elisha, saying, "Your servant my husband is dead, and you know that your servant feared the LORD. And the creditor is coming to take my two sons to be his slaves" (2 Kings 4:1).

A Woman: This story is about a woman. This story is about the church. In scripture a woman represents the church. Support for this is found in Jeremiah and Isaiah. "I have likened the daughter of Zion to a lovely and delicate woman" (Jeremiah 6:2). "For your Maker *is* your husband, The LORD of hosts *is* His name; He is called the God of the whole earth" (Isaiah 54:5).

Christ is the Bridegroom and Husband and the church is His bride. Parables in the New Testament support this concept as well. See: Matthew 9:15, Mark 2:19,20; Luke 5:34,35; and Matthew 25:1-11.

Certain Woman: This would indicate that this story is not just about the church at large; although, it can certainly have a universal application. This story is primarily about a problem that occurs in the local church. As we shall see it is a story about problems that occur in every church.

Cried Out: This is an indication of distress. This is a church in trouble. Churches today have numerous problems. Many churches are experiencing falling membership, diminished attendance at services, plummeting offerings and a general lack of vitality. What is the problem in the local church?

Husband Is Dead: Christ is the husband of the church. This passage indicates that Christ who is the husband of the church has died. Christ did die. Christ's death has created a problem, which is actually a challenge and opportunity for the church.

This passage might also indicate the attitude of some churches today. Christ may no longer be the living, energizing force in the church. Some churches languish in formalism and meaningless rounds of religious activities. To such a church, Christ is still dead.

Creditor: A creditor is someone to whom you owe something. In this case, the death of the husband created a debt for this woman. This means that the death of Christ has created a debt for the church. What debt could this mean?

Paul understood that the death of Christ made him a debtor. "I am a debtor both to Greeks and to barbarians, both to wise and to unwise. So, as much as is in me, I am ready to preach the gospel to you who are in Rome also" (Romans 1:14, 15).

The debt the church owes is to both the Greeks and barbarians, both to wise and unwise. In other words, the whole world. But in a local sense, your local church owes a debt to your community, your neighbors and friends.

Your community has a right to ask, "What role are you playing in the life of the community? Justify yourself. Show us that you are worthy of a place in our community. What are you doing for us? How are you helping us? How are you an asset rather than a liability?"

These are the questions every local church must answer for herself. The community has a right to know who you are, why you exist in the community and what your business is. You and your local church owe a debt to your community.

Two Sons: The two sons represent church members. The two indicates that there are two classes of people in the church. The following texts are about two sons and refer to the different experiences of church members. "But what do you think? A man had two sons, and he came to the first and said, 'Son, go, work today in my vineyard.' He answered and said, 'I will not,' but afterward he regretted it and went. Then he came to the second and said likewise. And he answered and said, 'I go, sir,' but he did not go. Which of the two did the will of his father?" They said to Him, "The first." Jesus said to them, "Assuredly, I say to you that tax collectors and harlots enter the kingdom of God before you" (Matthew 21:28-31).

In this passage is the contrast between talkers and doers. Some in the church talk a good story but don't do much. There are others who quietly go about the business of doing good.

> "Then He said: 'A certain man had two sons. And the younger of them said to his father, 'Father, give me the portion of goods that falls to me.' So he divided to them his livelihood. And not many days after, the younger son gathered all together, journeyed to a far country, and there wasted his possessions with prodigal living. But when he had spent all, there arose a severe famine in that land, and he began to be in want. Then he went and joined himself to a citizen of that country, and he sent him into his fields to feed swine. And he would gladly have filled his stomach with the pods that the swine ate, and no one gave him anything.
>
> 'But when he came to himself, he said, 'How many of my father's hired servants have bread enough and to spare, and I perish with hunger! I will arise and go to my father, and will say to him, "Father, I have sinned against heaven and before you, and I am no longer worthy to be called your son. Make me like one of your hired servants."'
>
> "And he arose and came to his father. But when he was still a great way off, his father saw him and had compassion, and ran and fell on his neck and kissed him. And the son said to him, 'Father, I have sinned against heaven and in your sight, and am no longer worthy to be called your son.'
>
> "But the father said to his servants, 'Bring out the best robe and put it on him, and put a ring on his hand and sandals on his feet. And bring the fatted calf here and kill it, and let us eat and be merry; for this my son was dead and is alive again; he was lost and is found.' And they began to be merry.
>
> "Now his older son was in the field. And as he came and drew near to the house, he heard music and dancing. So he called one of the servants and asked what these things meant. And he said to him, 'Your brother has come, and because he has received him safe and sound, your father has killed the fatted calf.'
>
> "But he was angry and would not go in. Therefore his father came out and pleaded with him. So he answered and said to his father, 'Lo, these many years I have been serving you; I never transgressed your commandment at any time;

and yet you never gave me a young goat, that I might make merry with my friends. But as soon as this son of yours came, who has devoured your livelihood with harlots, you killed the fatted calf for him.'

"And he said to him, 'Son, you are always with me, and all that I have is yours. It was right that we should make merry and be glad, for your brother was dead and is alive again, and was lost and is found'"(Luke 15:11-32).

This is the familiar story of the prodical son and the older brother. Each son represents a different type of church member. In this story, both boys were lost. One in the church and the other in a far country. -

"For it is written that Abraham had two sons: the one by a bondwoman, the other by a freewoman" (Galatians 4:22).

Here again two sons represent different types of church members. Some are still in bondage as represented by Ishmael and the others are free because they have been born again. These types of church members are represented by Isaac.

Slaves: It is the creditor that is coming to make slaves of this woman's sons. The world is coming to make slaves of church members. The church is daily being converted to the world. We see members drifting into sin. Compromise within the church is rampant. Church members are becoming slaves to fashion. Church members are becoming slaves to appetite. Church members are becoming slaves to alcohol. Church members are becoming slaves to entertainment and ease.

The church might well cry out in distress for the loss of her members. The world has come and has stolen the hearts and minds of many church members. This is the condition of the Laodicean church which exactly describes the condition of the church today.

2 Kings 4:2

Now let us look at 2 Kings 4:2 to see the problem develop further.

"So Elisha said to her, "What shall I do for you? Tell me, what do you have in the house?" And she said, "Your maidservant has nothing in the house but a jar of oil" (2 Kings 4:2).

Elisha: This is the prophet who was the spiritual leader of his day and symbolically represents the authority of the church. Elisha represents church administration at its various levels. It is natural for the local church to turn to the conference administration for help in times of distress. Elisha represents the ecclesiastical authority of the church. Let us notice the response given to the cry of distress from the local church. I have divided the response into two parts.

What Shall I Do for You? This indicates some limitation on the part of church authority. Just as the Christian experience of one person cannot substitute for another; just so, the church authorities cannot compensate for any deficits to be found in your congregation. The role of church authority is primarily advisory. Church leaders may counsel with us and pray with us and study the problem with us but in the end the local church still has the problem and has to be the organization to do something about the problem.

What do You Have in The House? This is a logical question. It calls for an inventory of resources. It asks, "What assets exist at the local level that can be utilized to help solve the problem?"

Your Maidservant Has Nothing: Now here is a dishonest assessment of the situation. This lady had two sons but didn't value them as highly as she should. She didn't mention them. Her sons should have been counted among her assets. And so it is today with local churches. The pastor is shouldered with too many of the responsibilities that should be carried by church members. The church members are less and less involved in the life of the church. There is very little life in many churches.

A Jar of Oil: I suspect this is a complaint rather than a boast. The lady only had a jar of oil. Oil in scripture represents the Holy Spirit. Anointing with oil was used to symbolize the anointing by the Holy Spirit. It is to be applied in the name of the Lord.

"I have found My servant David; With My holy oil I have anointed him"(Psalm 89:20).

"Is anyone among you sick? Let him call for the elders of the church, and let them pray over him, anointing him with oil in the name of the Lord" (James 5:14).

This connection between oil and the Holy Spirit is mentioned in Testimonies To Ministers in the following passage.

> "Read and study the fourth chapter of Zechariah. The two olive trees empty the golden oil out of themselves through the golden pipes into the golden bowl from which the lamps of the sanctuary are fed. *The golden oil represents the Holy Spirit.* With this oil God's ministers are to be constantly supplied, that they, in turn, may impart it to church. "Not by might, nor by power, but by My Spirit, saith the Lord of hosts." Testimonies to Ministers and Gospel Workers 188

Oil Creates Light: Let's examine the role of oil a bit more. It was used in lamps to create light. What does light represent?

Light Represents Good Works: In the following passages you will see that light, the product of the Holy Spirit in the life, represents good works. "Let your light so shine before men, that they may see your good works and glorify your Father in heaven"(Matthew 5:16). In this next passage is described the work of health evangelism.

> "Is this not the fast that I have chosen:
> To loose the bonds of wickedness,
> To undo the heavy burdens,
> To let the oppressed go free,
> And that you break every yoke?
> Is it not to share your bread with the hungry,
> And that you bring to your house the poor who are cast out;
> When you see the naked, that you cover him,
> And not hide yourself from your own flesh?
> Then your light shall break forth like the morning,
> Your healing shall spring forth speedily,
> And your righteousness shall go before you;
> The glory of the LORD shall be your rear guard.
> If you extend your soul to the hungry
> And satisfy the afflicted soul,
> Then your light shall dawn in the darkness,
> And your darkness shall *be* as the noonday" (Isaiah 58:6-8, 10).

Helping people stop smoking, eat right, lose weight and exercise are all comprehended in loosening the bonds of wickedness, undoing heavy burdens, and letting the oppressed go free. Isaiah 58 describes health evangelism. Health evangelism is good works and it results in light.

The lady in this story was low on oil. This symbolically means that this local church was low on the presence and influence of the Holy Spirit. It was a cold and lifeless church with members disappearing out the back door. This church was deficient in good works. The members were not involved in any outreach activities. They didn't have a health evangelism program. Now let's look at the advice Elisha gave in this crisis situation.

2 Kings 4:3

"Then he said, "Go, borrow vessels from everywhere, from all your neighbors—empty vessels; do not gather just a few." (2 Kings 4:3).

Go: Here is beginning of the solution to the problem. The word is "GO." This means get busy. Do something. It represents action. The problem in the local church is a lack of action. The answer to the problem in the local church is activity. Start to do something. The instruction doesn't stop here. Very specific instruction is given.

Borrow Vessels: Vessels in scripture represent people as confirmed by the following passages from the Old and New Testaments.

"But in a great house there are not only vessels of gold and silver, but also of wood and clay, some for honor and some for dishonor. Therefore if anyone cleanses himself from the latter, *he will be a vessel* for honor, sanctified and useful for the Master, prepared for every good work" (2 Timothy 2:20,21).

"And the vessel that he made of clay was marred in the hand of the potter; so he made it again into another vessel, as it seemed good to the potter to make.

"O house of Israel, can I not do with you as this potter?" says the LORD. "Look, as the clay is in the potter's hand, so are you in My hand, O house of Israel! (Jeremiah 18:4,6).

"I am forgotten like a dead man, out of mind; I am like a broken vessel". (Psalm 31:12).

The vessels are to be borrowed. They are not to be stolen or bought but borrowed. Borrowing is an act of asking. In our work with those whose lives are to be changed by health evangelism we are to invite and ask. We want to borrow them for a few days to introduce them to God who has the power to change their lives. No force is to be used in the work of God.

The word "GO" indicated that action was necessary. We have next established that the action was to involve people. Next we learn the scope of the work.

Everywhere, from all your neighbors: The activities of the local church are to involve neighbors. This indicates that the local church is supposed to do a work in its own community. Oh, yes, you need to give to missions and radio and TV ministries but the biggest work is right among your neighbors.

ALL neighbors are included in the instruction. All neighbors are to be the field of labor. But there is a certain restriction which is placed on the selection of a neighbor to be served. There is a form of discrimination and exclusiveness which is to be practiced. The labor is to be confined to *empty* vessels.

Empty vessels: Empty vessels represent people who feel empty. These are not the proud, egotistical people who are brimming with self-esteem. These are not people who think they have a power within themselves that will propel them to success. No, the empty vessels are those who realize their own weakness. They have tried to succeed on their own but have found their own efforts to be inadequate. These are the ones who are hungering and thirsting after righteousness. Our health evangelism activities should be confined to those who want help.

Do not borrow just a few: Here is a reminder of the scope of activity. The local church in its activities is not to be contented with feeble, intermittent, or spasmodic efforts. The church is to reach every interested and eligible person in the community.

The admonition to do a thorough work is emphasized three times in this one verse with the words, "everywhere," "all your neighbors" and "do not gather a few."

And now the prescription for success continues in the next verse.

2 Kings 4:4

"And when you have come in, you shall shut the door behind you and your sons; then pour it into all those vessels, and set aside the full ones" (2 Kings 4:4)

When you have come in, you shall shut the door behind you. Come in where? In the house of this woman. Of course the house is the church building itself. Here is a strong indication that the major emphasis in any Holy Spirit related activity is to be IN the church itself. This is why I don't like to conduct health evangelism in any other setting than the church. The church is the Christian's home. The sooner a person gets there the better off he or she will be.

If we spend all our time conducting health evangelism in high school auditoriums or other public places, the church doesn't get the recognition, church members don't help and people don't get into the church. It is hard to get people into the local church for traditional doctrinal presentations but it is *not* difficult to get people to come to your local church for health evangelism activities. The church is designated by this scripture as the place for evangelistic activity.

I think this is also indicated by the shutting the door behind you. In this story a very special miracle is about to take place and it only occurs in connection with the church. The church is God's appointed agency for the salvation of the world. This activity is to take place in the church.

Then pour into all those vessels: Here is where the advice seems illogical. This woman only had a jar of oil. How is she going to pour out into ALL those vessels? If she put a teaspoon of oil in each vessel, she wouldn't have enough to go around. If she poured a jar full into just one big vessel she would only be able to recover a small amount if she tried to get it all back.

In God's instruction as to how we should work and what we should do there is always room for doubt, questioning and speculation. The instruction given here seems unrealistic and unreasonable but it is very specific and it is clear. Here is where faith is to be exercised.

The pouring out is especially significant and needs some further explanation. The goal here is to fill the vessels with oil which is synonymous with filling people with the holy spirit. The miracle is only going to occur when the pouring begins. This lady didn't want to lose the little bit of oil she did have. She could have placed the jar of oil on a board that stretched across the opening of a 50-gallon drum and could have prayed for God to cause the jar to overflow with oil so that the little bit she had wouldn't be risked at all.

In other words, the lady could have asked or prayed for an abundance of the oil to spill over the sides of the jar. She could have asked for oil above and beyond the small amount she had, without risking her own pitifully small supply.

This is a critical principle in spreading the Gospel. The Holy Spirit is dispensed by God in proportion to our efforts to work in God's cause in spreading the Good News. If we don't give away what we have we never get any more. If you have too little of the Holy Spirit in your local church, the key to getting an abundant outpouring from God is not found in praying for more of the Holy Spirit but to start doing something with the pitifully small amount you have.

This principle is made perfectly clear in these selected passages.

> "The capacity for receiving the holy oil from the two olive trees which empty themselves, is by the receiver emptying that holy oil out of himself in word and in action to supply the necessities of other souls. Work, precious, satisfying work—to be constantly receiving and constantly imparting! *The capacity for receiving is only kept up by imparting* (NL No. 12, pp. 3, 4). S.D.A. Bible Commentary Vol. 4, p.1180.

> "Our mission to the world is not to serve or please ourselves; we are to glorify God by co-operating with Him to save sinners. We are to ask blessings from God that we may communicate to others. *The capacity for receiving is preserved only by imparting.* We cannot continue to receive heavenly treasure without communicating to those around us. Christ's Object Lessons, 142-143.

Church members are like pipes through which the Holy Spirit flows to others. If the faucet is shut off nothing will flow through the pipe. If the spigot is open there is flow. You may be just a small section of pipe in the plumbing of the church but there is an unlimited amount of the Holy Spirit that can flow through you to bless others.

Set aside the full ones: Is there ever a sense that we set aside those for whom we are working? Certainly! As soon as people have become filled with the Holy Spirit and their lives have been changed, it is time to set them beside us so they can help us work for others. This is not setting aside people just to get them out of the way. It is that we no longer need to work over them because they themselves are now filled with the Holy Spirit and are enabled to impart the Holy Spirit to others themselves.

As soon as a person has been converted it is time to put them to work. There is something they can do. They should be part of a team so they won't work independently or unwisely.

> "Just as soon as a church is organized, the members should be set to work, taught to go forth in God-given power to find others and tell them of the story of redeeming love. The power of the gospel is to come upon the companies raised up, fitting them for service. Some of the *new converts* will be so filled with the power of the Lord that they will *at once enter the work*, imparting that which they have received." Manuscript Releases Volume Five, 331.

> "I saw that the servants of God should not go over and over the same field of labor, but should be searching out souls in new places. Those who are already established in the truth should not demand so much of their labor; for they *ought to be able to stand alone*, and strengthen others about them, while the messengers of God visit the dark and lonely places, setting the truth before those who are not now enlightened as to the present truth." Early Writings of Ellen G. White, 104.

Now for the results of this story.

2 Kings 4:5

"So she went from him and shut the door behind her and her sons, who brought the vessels to her; and she poured it out"(2 Kings 4:5)

So she went: This is the correct response. The advice was, "Go." So she went. We know from the previous verses that this corrective activity occurred behind closed doors in the church. Notice the next phrase.

Her sons, who brought the vessels to her: Here is a surprise. The work of bringing people into the church is not the work of the pastor. It is the work of church members. This is why health evangelism activities aren't designed correctly unless they are designed to create an interface between church members and the public.

This one-on-one interaction between the sons of the woman, (church members) and the empty vessels, occurs in the setting of the church.

And she poured out: This represents activity for the lost. For those who have spiritual needs, those who have physical needs and those who have bad habits and addictions. They can change their behavior once they have a relationship with God and are filled with the Holy Spirit. This occurs in the church with a wide variety of health evangelism programs.

2 Kings 4:6

"Now it came to pass, when the vessels were full, that she said to her son, "Bring me another vessel." And he said to her, "There is not another vessel." So the oil ceased (2 Kings 4:6).

Now it came to pass: There is a lot we need to understand in these few words. The work of God in the earth takes time. Time, effort and means are required. We should not become weary in doing good.

"Bring me another vessel": What a change has taken place in this woman! At the beginning of this story she was crying and worried about the state of her home, and family. Now this woman is excited. She likes the work she is doing. The work is satisfying and effective. It is enjoyable. When the work appears to be done and there are no more vessels to be filled she urges her sons to "Bring me another vessel."

Health evangelism and associated working for souls is a very exciting and satisfying work. The more you do the more you want to do. It is exciting to see lives changed through the wonder-working power of the Holy Spirit. Start doing health evangelism and you will create an excited, vibrant church that loves to reach out to the community.

"There is not another vessel": This indicates that the sons of this woman did a thorough work. They were busy. They scoured the neighborhood to find empty vessels. The work didn't cease until everyone who was empty was filled. And so it will be in the last days. The gospel must go to every kindred, tongue and nation. It will largely be done one community at a time. But there is an end to the work. Once everyone who is going to make a decision to follow God does so, the will be finished.

So the oil ceased: How comforting to know that there will be enough oil until every empty vessel is filled. There will be enough converting power of the Holy Spirit until all have decided one way or another. The oil will cease some day. That day is spoken of in Matthew and Revelation.

"And this gospel of the kingdom will be preached in all the world as a witness to all the nations, and then the end will come" (Matthew 24:14).

"He who is unjust, let him be unjust still; he who is filthy, let him be filthy still; he who is righteous, let him be righteous still; he who is holy, let him be holy still."(Revelation 22:11).

The reward follows.

2 Kings 4:7

"Then she came and told the man of God. And he said, "Go, sell the oil and pay your debt; and you and your sons live on the rest." (2 Kings 4:7)

Pay your debt: Let's see if we can make sense of this last passage. How can anything we do actually pay our debt? Our debt was paid once and for all on Calvary. The abundance of oil that was produced through this miracle was in no way the property of the widow. It was God's oil and how could that in any way pay her debt?

Actually, the debt mentioned here is not the "eternal debt" we owe our Saviour but the debt we owe our friends and neighbors. In our working for them we do gain reward. Stars in our crowns and a hearty "Well done" from Jesus at his second coming. "His lord said to him, 'Well done, good and faithful servant; you were faithful over a few things, I will make you ruler over many things. Enter into the joy of your lord.'" (Matthew 25:21).

And live: The gift of God is eternal life but we cooperate with Him in working for the betterment and salvation of our neighbors and friends. This then is the Biblical model of health evangelism. Church members working out of the local church in the surrounding neighborhood finding people in need and providing whatever services they can and pointing to God as the agent of behavior change in our human life.

"These are words which Christ addresses to his redeemed people. He invites them to become patient toilers in a field which calls for self-denying labor; but it is a glorious work, and one that Heaven smiles upon. *Faithful work is more acceptable to God than the most zealous formal worship.* True worship consists in working together with Christ. Prayers, exhortations, and talk are cheap fruits, which are frequently tied on; but fruits that are manifested in good works, in caring for the needy, the fatherless, and widows, are genuine, and grow naturally upon a good tree. The Signs of the Times 02-17-1887

Summary

1. The church is having problems. Members are being taken over by the world.

2. The church is to be a focal point of activity.

3. Church members are to do the work.

4. The Holy Spirit will energize our activities but only after we get to work with what we have.

5. This is exciting, soul-winning work that will occur until Christ comes.

6. There will be a "well done" for good and faithful servants.

11

As Solid as Science

Science and religion are mutually exclusive disciplines in the minds of some; but, the role of science in health evangelism is an important one. Science has done much to advance our standard of living and has provided us with wonderful technologies. The scientific method is an invaluable tool that can validate or discredit the effectiveness of a drug or health practice. Traditional religious evangelism deals primarily with a person's spiritual condition. Health evangelism deals with both spiritual and physical restoration. The tools of science are essential to measure the effectiveness of health evangelism.

In the area of healthful living, science and evangelism are both important. Science provides the proof that certain health practices preserve health and promote long life. Health evangelism introduces us to God who provides us with the ability to change who we are and gives us the strength to do what is best for our health.

The Scientific Method

The scientific method is the tool that science uses to prove a point. The scientific method is extremely valuable and is responsible for establishing the validity and effectiveness of drugs, healthful practices, and a whole host of technological advances. Science proved that cigarette smoking caused lung cancer and science put robots on Mars.

As you conduct health evangelism activities, it is important to use ideas and data that are scientifically sound. Selecting accurate information will be easy for someone with a scientific background but will be a challenge for those not trained in the scientific method.

I want to introduce you to some tools that are used by science which you should consider when gathering and sorting out information for use in your health evangelism programs. I am concerned with those procedures used to collect and analyze data. Every recommendation for healthful living should be tested and proven effective in a human population. You need to be able to look for scientific articles that support what you are telling people. You should be able to analyze a study to see if it was done in such a way as to be able to really prove a point.

Anecdotal Reports and Endorsements

The most useless and unscientific recommendations for a product, diet, nutritional supplement or proposed lifestyle change is the anecdotal report. When there is no science to back up a claim of effectiveness for a product, you can at least get someone to recommend it. You frequently see the claim, "I tried this for 10 days and I feel so much better." This is merely an advertising ploy and not scientific evidence.

I have seen full page advertisements for products with as many as a dozen endorsements by people who have been benefitted by the use of some pill. Endorsements do not establish the validity of anything. When you want to include some new element in a health evangelism program, make sure it is based on sound science and avoid any product or concept if the only proof of effectiveness is the anecdotal reports of those who use the product.

How The Supplement Was Made

Using scientific techniques to produce a nutritional supplement isn't good enough. I have seen claims that a certain pill was created in the most carefully controlled environment. The plants used in the pills were cultivated under strict environmental conditions. The plants were harvested at the peak of maturity. The leaves were processed in an accurate manner. The pills were filled under exacting conditions of cleanliness and with scientific exactness. All of this care in production is important but doesn't mean that this pill will do anything for you.

Do Pills Work?

The scientific method has been highly developed to study this question. The pharmaceutical industry is regulated by the Food and Drug Administration (FDA) of the United States Government. Rigorous requirements are imposed on anyone who seeks official approval for a new drug. It can cost over $100 million to bring a new drug to market. The expense is due to the rigorous scientific method that must be applied to the study of new drugs.

On the other hand, the FDA does not provide any significant oversight to those pills that are sold as "dietary supplements." One could powder pansy petals and promote them as a nutritional supplement that preserves prostate health. You could advertise and sell these capsules without any government approval. The cost would be low and the profit high. But do powdered pansy petals really help the prostate? You won't know unless you do the kind of science required by the FDA for regular pharmaceuticals.

If you have an idea that some food extract will cure or prevent some disease it would be easiest to first study the product in an animal model. You start by finding a species of animal that has a disease similar to that found in humans. If your powdered pansy petal pill was shown to benefit diseased animals and did not injure or kill them from toxic side effects, then it would be time to try your pills out on real people.

There are so many biases that can creep into studies that they must be carefully controlled for or eliminated. One way to do this is with a *control group*. Your new, powerful, health promoting product needs to be compared with a *placebo*. This will prove if your drug is better or worse than nothing. You can't put the placebo in a white pill but the test drug in a red pill because this would create an unfair bias in favor of the red pill. To be fair and accurate the placebo and the test drug need to be presented in exactly the same form. Both the control group getting the placebo and the test group getting the real drug need to get the same number of the same color of pills at the same time every day.

Another bias could result from doctors who might know the real drug from the placebo and could record favorable results for the test drug in their reports. For this reason the doctor prescribing a test drug needs to be ignorant of whether he or she is prescribing the real drug or the placebo. If a study is designed so the patient doesn't know what he or she is getting the study is said to be *blinded*. If the prescribing doctor also doesn't know what he or she is prescribing then the study is *double blinded*.

Another way to control for bias is to switch the real drug back and forth between the two groups of test patients. In this way the placebo group would get the real drug after six weeks or six months of placebo and the test group would get the placebo after six weeks or six months of the real drug. When this element is added to a study, it is called a *cross over* study.

The best kind of study to prove the effectiveness of a test product is a double blinded cross over study. These kinds of studies take time, cost a lot of money, and have ethical implications. They are conducted under the watchful eye of an institutional peer review committee which has ultimate authority whether a researcher can initiate, continue or needs to terminate a study.

Virtually none of the nutritional supplements that crowd store shelves have been studied in this way. For this reason, the claims made for most supplements are claims which have not been substantiated by rigorous scientific study. The efficacy of a nutritional supplement or drug is established by the scientific method. If you are considering promoting some pill as part of a health evangelism program look for data from double blind cross over studies as proof of the pill's effectiveness. Favorable testimonials by recognizable actors or athletes don't carry any scientific weight.

Side effects

Side effects are temporary symptoms or long term adverse outcomes produced by the ingestion or application of a product. Side effects may be mild or severe. Knowing the expected side effects of a drug or nutritional supplement is important. Side effects may include nausea, vomiting, diarrhea, skin rash, or itching. More severe side effects might include liver or kidney damage. An extreme side effect may result in death.

When a drug is being studied, patients receiving the placebo and the test drug are given long questionnaires to find out what they are feeling as they take the medication (or the placebo). Symptoms that could be side effects are carefully documented. The researchers then compare the side effects attributed to the placebo with the side effects that result from the test drug. Most test subjects will report some side effects to both the test drug and the placebos. The placebo should ideally produce no side effects as it is usually filled with a small amount of sugar, starch or cellulose.

Because patients know they are enrolled in a test study, they are more sensitive to small changes in their body which they may attribute to the drug or the placebo. If a study showed that 10 percent of people taking the placebo got nauseated and 15 percent of the people taking the test drug got nausea, you could correctly assume that the test drug caused nausea at a rate 5% above that of the placebo.

Nutritional supplement packages don't usually list any side effects on the label or in promotional materials. This is because most supplements have never been tested for side effects. The usual claim is that because a product is "all natural" that there will be no side effects. I would point out that tobacco is "all natural" and it kills over 450,000 U.S. citizens every year. Arsenic is natural and it will kill you. Mercury is natural and it causes serious toxic effects. Salt is natural but can lead to high blood pressure. All food supplements will cause some kind of side effects in some people. We don't know what the side effects are because the manufactures of food supplements are not required to study or publish the side effects caused by their products.

Do not promote products in any of your health evangelism program unless you know that the product has been specifically tested for side effects compared to a placebo. Do not accept the statement that it is a natural "food supplement" and cannot have any side effects. All foods and supplements have some side effects in some people.

Safety

Safety is related to side effects. Side effects may disappear when a drug or supplement is stopped. Some drugs and supplements may cause more serious or even permanent damage to a person's health. Ephedra was a component of several popular weight loss supplements that were sold over the counter. After several cardiac deaths were reported with the use of Ephedra containing products the FDA stepped in and banned the use of this substance in supplements of all kinds.

Many licensed drugs have safety issues. Often these are outweighed by the benefits that occur in critical situations. The drugs that are used to cure lymphoma cancer will cause a drop in your red cells causing anemia, your hair will fall out and other serious problems can develop. These are serious safety problems but are usually temporary and disappear after your cancer treatment is over. Of course, on the other hand, you will die of a lymphoma if it isn't treated and serious safety problems with the cancer drugs are acceptable because your life is at stake.

You just don't know what serious safety issues are involved with a food supplement unless that product is tested. Within a 6-month period, I had two patients in my private practice of medicine who presented with liver failure caused by dietary supplements they were taking. These products had no warnings of any kinds on their labels. Fortunately, in each case, the liver abnormalities promptly resolved after the offending supplement was stopped.

Do not promote or sell supplements in your health evangelism program. If program participants seem particularly interested in some product, check to see if it has been tested in a double-blind, crossover, placebo-controlled study that looked at side effects and generated safety data. Claims are not enough. Look at the study design. Look at the numbers of people involved and the duration of the study. Almost all nutritional supplements have not been subjected to this type of analysis.

Population Studies

The effectiveness of medications can be studied in fairly small populations. Much larger studies are needed to document the benefits or harm from specific lifestyle behaviors. If someone promotes a certain behavior as important to health, it is important for you to learn what you can about the population in which that behavior was studied. Often, studies are just surveys of opinions. Perhaps a few dozen people were polled. Such studies don't prove anything.

The simplest form population of study is the *retrospective* study. A retrospective study starts with a population that has a certain disease. The researcher then collects data from a second population of people who do not have that disease. The more alike the two populations are in every respect except for the presence of disease, the more valid the conclusions that can be drawn.

In a retrospective study the two populations should be matched for age. You wouldn't want one population to be older than the other as many diseases increase with age. The two populations should be matched for sex. You wouldn't want to compare a population of men with a population of women because many diseases are more common in men than women and of course the opposite is true as well. You would want the two populations to be from the same geographic area. If a study group was from an urban area, you shouldn't compare that population with a group of people who live in a rural setting as many health problems are different in different geographical locations.

Careful matching of case and control populations is the most important part of a retrospective study. Inaccurate results can occur if care is not taken in the selection of a control group. In the 1950's it was several retrospective studies of men with lung cancer that showed that smoking cigarettes was a much more common behavior in men with lung cancer than in a matched control group of men who did not have lung cancer. Retrospective studies are most useful in studying rather rare diseases. As far as population studies go, retrospective studies are relatively inexpensive to conduct. Many retrospective studies are conducted with a hundred cases and a hundred controls.

The *prospective* population study is an even better scientific tool. Prospective population studies are conducted on large populations of people and are continued for several years. We are talking of enrolling thousands to even millions of people. In a prospective study, you start by enrolling people by administering a questionnaire that determines a wide variety of behaviors. You collect basic data regarding age, sex, race, occupation. You ask about the daily or weekly use of various food items. You ask about alcohol, tobacco and drug use. You ask about levels of exercise at work and at home.

You might want to do certain physical measurements such as height, weight, blood pressure, cholesterol levels or other physical parameters. You usually exclude people with known diseases so that you can measure the effect of certain behaviors in healthy people.

Prospective studies take a long time to conduct. You have to run them for enough years for diseases to develop and deaths to occur. You periodically monitor the health of the population and document the development of disease over time.

The American Cancer Society has conducted large prospective studies that have enrolled over one million people and has followed the subjects for several years. A large Japanese study followed over 250,000 people for some 17 years. A large prospective study can be used to study the development of many different diseases that may be associated with many different behaviors. The Framingham heart study enrolled only 4000 people but followed them for more than 30 years.

The most valid data regarding various behaviors and health come from prospective studies. Many claims are made for many different health behaviors but if there isn't data from prospective studies to back up the claims don't put a lot of stock in what is being claimed.

Prospective studies were the first to show that cigarette smoking was not only a cause of lung cancer but was also a major cause of cancers at other sites as well. Smoking causes cancer of the oral cavity, larynx, esophagus, pancreas, kidney, bladder and cervix. Smoking causes emphysema and chronic bronchitis. Smoking is a major cause of heart attacks, strokes, and hardening of the arteries in general. All of these facts were discovered in several large prospective studies. One large prospective study can prove several things.

Other prospective studies have shown that you can prevent heart attacks by: eating nuts frequently, drinking four or more glasses of water a day and by decreasing the amount of meat and dairy products in the diet. Don't believe a health claim unless there is some objective data from a large prospective study.

Peer Review and Publication

Most manufactures of nutritional supplements promote their products through attractively produced pamphlets, videos or DVDs. The same people that make the pills, sell the pills. There is no process of keeping them honest except through oversight by the FDA or peer review.

Research regarding drugs or populations have a time-honored mechanism to keep things honest. It is the *peer review* process. Research at every center of scientific study is monitored by a peer review committee. Any bias in study design or population selection is pretty much eliminated through the peer review process.

Peer review continues when it comes time to publish research data. Scientists are not allowed to produce slick promotional pieces for the products they produce. Research is introduced to the world through publication in a respected medical journal. The author must reveal the product, its chemical structure, the population in which it was tested, the design of the study and the results including side effects.

The editors of scientific journals distribute the articles they receive for publication to several independent (often competing) scientists who are doing research in the same area. If the study was sound and the results accurate, the article is recommended for publication. If defects or inaccuracies are found, the article is returned to the author for clarification, revision or perhaps more research is needed to adequately prove the point.

Do not promote or sell supplements, report on research, or promote certain behaviors unless everything is supported by articles in the peer-reviewed scientific literature. The medical literature of the entire world is catalogued in the National Library of Medicine in Bethesda, Maryland. Authors, article title, journal, and a brief abstract is published on line. The articles from over 5000 different medical journals are catalogued each month and are available for review on line. A variety of library services are available online at nlm.nih.gov/. This is where all relevant health articles can be located. Hard copies of articles can be ordered online or obtained through your local library.

Do not promote any health concept, idea or practice in your health evangelism program unless you can find support for it in multiple places in peer-reviewed scientific articles. Every health activity promoted in your health evangelism program should be supported by sound scientific evidence.

The Bible supports this type of rigorous accuracy in all we do. "Let all things be done decently and in order, 1 Corinthians 14:40." The Old and New Testaments contain dozens of recommendations to be orderly in all that we do.

Spirit of Prophecy Comments on Science

In this quotation Mrs. White correctly identifies science with all kinds of power. Science is useful. Accurate science should be a part of any health evangelism program.

> "The schools established among us are matters of grave responsibility; for important interests are involved. In a special manner our schools are a spectacle unto angels and to men. *A knowledge of science of all kinds is power*, and it is in the purpose of God that advanced science shall be taught in our schools as a preparation for the work that is to precede the closing scenes of earth's history. The truth is to go to the remotest bounds of the earth, through agents trained for the work. But while the knowledge of science is a power, the knowledge which Jesus in person came to impart to the world was the knowledge of the gospel. The light of truth was to flash its bright rays into the uttermost parts of the earth, and the acceptance or rejection of the message of God involved the eternal destiny of souls." Fundamentals of Christian Education 186

In this next quotation, a practical knowledge of the science of human life is advocated. This knowledge has been produced through many hundreds of thousands of scientific research studies conducted over the past 100 years.

> "Children are sent to school to be taught the sciences; but the science of human life is wholly neglected. That which is of the most vital importance, a true knowledge of themselves, without which all other science can be of but little advantage, is not brought to their notice. A cruel and wicked ignorance is tolerated in regard to this important question. So closely is health related to our happiness that we cannot have the latter without the former. *A practical knowledge of the science of human life, is necessary in order to glorify God in our bodies.* It is therefore of the highest importance that among the studies selected for childhood, physiology should occupy the first place. How few know anything about the structure and functions of their own bodies, and of Nature's laws. Many are drifting about without knowledge, like a ship at sea without compass or anchor; and what is more, they are not interested to learn how to keep their bodies in a healthy condition, and prevent disease." The Health Reformer 08-01-1866

Lectures for the public should contain the science of health and Christian temperance. In this next quotation there is a call for scientific knowledge and accuracy in all public presentations.

"The Lord has a message for our cities, and this message we are to proclaim in our camp-meetings, and by other public efforts, and also through our publications. In addition to this, hygienic restaurants are to be established in the cities, and by them the message of temperance is to be proclaimed. Arrangements should be made to hold meetings in connection with our restaurants. Whenever possible, let a room be provided where the patrons can be invited to *lectures on the science of health and Christian temperance*, where they can receive instruction on the preparation of wholesome food, and on other important subjects." Testimonies Vol. 7, p. 115.

Summary

1. The value of various health practices is established by sound science.

2. The scientific method is a useful tool in studying the field of health.

3. Effectiveness of a product requires scientific study.

4. Side effects and safety of health products must be determined.

5. Population studies are required to firmly establish the validity of a health concept.

6. Peer review and publication help establish the credibility of health concepts.

7. Scripture and the Spirit of Prophecy support sound science.

12

The Program is Not the End!

Follow-up has been the weakest component in all the health evangelism programs I have seen or have conducted; yet it is as important as the program itself. Follow-up is much different from conducting the program. It is more time consuming. It takes continuous effort and planning. There are some easy ways to attempt follow-up that aren't very effective.

In planning to include follow-up activities in a health evangelism program it is important to inform the small group partners that you require their help for follow-up activities as well as their help during the program. The time commitment required of a partner during the program is significant. The time commitment required for follow-up is still significant and requires more creativity and will occur at least quarterly for a period of one year. When church members are recruited, they should know up front that their services will be required for at least a year.

The easiest follow-up activities could be conducted at the church. At the last session of any program there is a spirit of fellowship and gratitude. People want the feeling to last. There is always a sincere desire to continue meeting on a regular basis for follow-up.

Just forget it. Follow-up meetings at the church do not work. The program is over. The participants can come back to the next program if they wish. They should be informed during the last two sessions of the current program as to when the next program is going to be conducted. They should be provided with advertising brochures for the next program to distribute to their family and friends.

If you decide to have follow-up meetings at the church, you will find that they are always poorly attended. There are two reasons why people don't return to follow-up meetings. One reason is that they are successful in maintaining their new behavior. This means they don't need follow-up meetings. They are doing just fine and feel no need to come.

134

The second reason people don't return to follow-up meetings at the church is they have relapsed into their old habits and addictions and are ashamed to return. So, whether your participants experience success or failure, few of them will ever return to follow-up meetings at the church. They are more likely to return to the next regular program for more encouragement or a second try if they have failed. It is also important to give your church members who were helpers and partners a rest. They worked hard during the program and need some time off to catch up on other things.

So, what kind of follow-up do you do if you don't have follow-up meetings in the church? You do house-to-house follow-up. You do one-on-one follow-up with the participants in their own homes. Many church members remember, often with some dread, the house-to-house work many churches used to do from year to year in the old "Harvest Ingathering" program. The annual ingathering program consisted of going from house to house soliciting funds for home and foreign missions.

The in-home follow-up contacts you will conduct following a health evangelism program are much different. These are not cold calls. You know the people you are calling upon. You saw these people from day to day and from week to week during the entire program. You are friends with these people.

The follow-up team should consist of two people. The most practical way to do this is for the two group partners who headed a group to be the ones to call on the members of their own little group. This means that they will only have to make six or seven calls to complete the first round of follow-up.

This in-home follow-up activity will not be a surprise to your program participants as they should have been informed that there was going to be a follow-up during the program. Your program participants will be expecting you to call. This is not a "cold" call. By-in-large the participants will be glad to see you.

There are several important reasons for doing your follow-up in the participants homes. One reason is to help reinforce the participants behavior change. A smoker will be less likely to relapse after a program if he or she knows you will be calling in the near future to encourage them and to check on their progress.

Another reason, is to document the long-term effectiveness of your health evangelism program. You are calling on each participant to document what they are doing. This information will go into the database and will measure the effectiveness of your program. This fulfills the scientific aspect of your program.

Scientific evaluation is the perfect "official" reason for a follow-up visit in the home. You are simply dropping by for data collection. That is nonthreatening and will not present a significant barrier to your home visit. You need to take a clipboard, pencil and follow-up forms with you. They should be in your hand when you knock on the door.

The most important reason for an in-home follow-up visit is that this is probably the very first time you will be one-on-one with an individual member of your small group. This creates a very private type of contact in which spiritual issues can be explored. I like to approach this in a direct but a nonthreatening manner. How do you go about setting this up?

The polite thing to do is to call ahead and make a definite appointment for a specific time to visit. In this way participants can have their houses in order and will not be embarrassed as they would be if you make an unannounced call. If you call for an appointment and the participant says that he or she would like to skip the follow-up visit you can ask if they would be willing to complete the follow-up questionnaire over the phone? The participant will always say, "Yes" and you can obtain your follow-up data over the phone. It should be noted in your database that the follow-up was a phone contact and not an in-person interview.

While you are on the phone, after the participant has answered the questions for the questionnaire you can then assume a more casual voice and make inquiry as to how the person is doing. I like to use the same approach whether I am in the home or conducting the interview over the phone.

How is the in-home visit structured? First you make the appointment in advance. You show up on time for the visit with your clipboard in hand. After initial casual comments you announce the desire to obtain information and then go ahead and ask the few questions. Then you put your clipboard down, sit back, relax and casually ask three more "unofficial" questions which should not appear to be related to the purpose of data collection at all.

The first question I ask is, "How are you doing physically since you…" (quit smoking or lost weight or finished the program)? The usual answer is, "Your program has helped me so much, etc."

The second question has to do with mental issues. I ask, "How are you doing mentally? Is it still a struggle? How are you keeping it up?"

The third question is the most important and that is "How are you doing spiritually with regard to your habit?" This is the *key moment* of your entire health evangelism program. You are one-on-one in the privacy of a person's home. There are no other group members watching or listening. If a participant is thinking about spiritual things, if they want to talk about what God is doing in their lives they will talk to you about it right now.

Health evangelism programs should be evangelistic. They are made evangelistic in the middle of the program when you explain the ways in which God helps with behavior change but health evangelism programs are MOST evangelistic when you ask a person about his or her personal relationship with God in the quietness of their own home.

What kind of responses will you get to this question? A common response is, "Oh, fine, just fine. What did you think about the football game last weekend?" This indicates a reluctance to speak to you directly about spiritual things. Don't press the point. These people think a lot of you and the health evangelism program. They are not offended that you brought up the subject since it was a part of your program which was conduced in the church.

Without a connection with God, participants aren't likely to maintain their new behavior very long. Perhaps the Holy Spirit will impress them to come to another program. Don't push the unwilling into a discussion of spiritual things.

Many however, will respond positively to your question about spiritual things. They will gladly confess that they are maintaining their behavior through a relationship with God. They will rejoice that they have a new and more practical understanding about what the Christian life is all about. They will praise your church for having such a practical religion that actually helps people with real problems.

Others will be anxious to know much more about your church. They will want to know about various things such as the Sabbath and other distinctive doctrines. I cannot tell you what to do next but you should be prepared for anything and everything. I like to keep a variety of pamphlets, Bible study lessons and several books and Bibles in the car to use under these circumstances. If a person expresses an interest in spiritual things and wants to begin a discussion with you be prepared.

It will not appear that this was the REAL reason you came calling because this discussion came after you obtained your scientific data. It will not appear that this was the REAL reason you came calling because you didn't bring in the religious material with you when you came in the door. You had to go back out to your car to get the EXTRA materials.

If you have a positive spiritual interaction with a group member it is important to offer a prayer before you leave the home. It is important for you to pray again in your car. Thank God for the developing spiritual relationship and ask for continued guidance as you continue your contact.

Follow-up activities should be initiated soon after the end of a program. I suggest at one month, three months, six months and a year. Most people who relapse do so fairly rapidly and an early follow-up will be helpful to your participants. There is room for flexibility here. You may want to conduct follow-up activities more frequently. Remember to negotiate this with your group partners who are largely responsible for follow-up.

If two partners can't go together for some reason, it may be necessary for the pastor, health professional or some other helper to go with one of the partners to call on the participants in their group. Remember, two-by-two is a Biblical principle and the way to go make these calls.

A follow-up newsletter is a good idea but not a substitute for the in-home visits. In a newsletter the success of various individuals can be reviewed, spiritual messages about overcoming can be included, and the dates for the next programs at the church can be announced.

Spirit of Prophecy Quotations on Follow-up Activities

Follow-up will result in baptisms.

> "For years light has been given upon this point, showing the necessity of following up an interest that has been raised, and in no case leaving it until all have decided that lean toward the truth, and have experienced the conversion necessary for baptism, and united with some church, or formed one themselves." Evangelism, 324.

If we don't do follow-up, the gains may unravel. This advice applies to health evangelism activities as well as to other ministerial activity.

> "I hope you will look at things candidly and not move impulsively or from feeling. Our ministers must be educated and trained to do their work more thoroughly. They should bind off the work and not leave it to ravel out. And they should look especially after the interests they have created, and not go away and never have any special interest after leaving a church. A great deal of this has been done." Evangelism, 324.

Follow-up activity is mandatory and not optional. This would apply to health evangelists as well as pastors.

> "There are no circumstances of sufficient importance to call a minister from an interest created by the presentation of truth. Even sickness and death are of less consequence than the salvation of souls for whom Christ made so immense a sacrifice. Those who feel the importance of the truth, and the value

of souls for whom Christ died, will not leave an interest among the people for any consideration. They will say, Let the dead bury their dead. Home interests, lands and houses, should not have the least power to attract from the field of labor." Evangelism, 324.

A follow-up letter can be mailed. Tracts and Bible study guides can be distributed at follow-up visits.

> "When at our large gatherings, make all the discourses highly reformative. Arouse the intellect. Bring up the talents possible into the efforts made, and then follow up the effort with tracts and pamphlets, with articles written in simple form, to make the subjects brought before them distinctly stated, that the word spoken may be repeated by the silent agent. Short, interesting articles should be arranged in cheap style, and scattered everywhere. They should be at hand upon every occasion where the truth is brought before the minds of those to whom it is new and strange." Counsels to Writers and Editors, 126.

Follow-up activities should be aggressive. It will be appropriate to chase people down under some circumstances. Don't give up.

> "We must not think of such a thing as discouragement, but hold fast to souls by the grasp of faith. Do not give up those for whom you are working. Go out in the mountains and seek the lost sheep. They may run from you, but you must follow them up, take them in your arms and bring them to Jesus. Pulpit effort should always be followed by personal labor. The worker must converse and pray with those who are concerned about their souls salvation. Those who listen to discourses should see in those who believe, an example in life and character that will make a deep impression upon them." The Home Missionary, February 1, 1890.

Medical missionaries are true evangelists. They should always go out two-by-two. This is especially important in urban areas.

> It is medical missionaries that are needed all through the field. Canvassers should improve every opportunity granted them to learn how to treat disease. Physicians should remember that they will often be required to perform the duties of a minister. Medical missionaries come under the head of evangelists. The workers should go forth two by two, that they may pray and consult together. Never should they be sent out alone. The Lord Jesus Christ sent forth His disciples two and two into all the cities of Israel. He gave them the commission, "Heal the sick that are therein, and say unto them, The kingdom of God is come nigh unto you." Medical Ministry, 249.

Follow-up creates the opportunity to take along pamphlets, Bible Study guides, and books which can be handed out when the chance comes up.

> "Now, when we go into the house we should not begin to talk of frivolous things, but come right to the point and say, I want you to love Jesus, for He has first loved you.... *Take along the publications* and ask them to read. When they see that you are sincere they will not despise any of your efforts. There is a way to reach the hardest hearts. Approach in the simplicity, and sincerity, and humility that will help us to reach the souls of them for whom Christ died." Welfare Ministry, 91.

We are to follow Christ's example and find our way to the fireside, with families in their own homes. This is so personal and creates opportunities for witness that won't come up in the health evangelism activity at the church.

> "To all who are working with Christ I would say, Wherever you can gain access to the people by the fireside, improve your opportunity. Take your Bible, and open before them its great truths. Your success will not depend so much upon your knowledge and accomplishments, as upon your ability to find your way to the heart. By being social and coming close to the people, you may turn the current of their thoughts more readily than by the most able discourse. The presentation of Christ *in the family, by the fireside, and in small gatherings in private houses,* is often more successful in winning souls to Jesus than are sermons delivered in the open air, to the moving throng, or even in halls or churches." Gospel Workers. (1915), 193

Follow-up in the home should not be for the purpose of doctrinal presentations but from time to time doctrinal issues will come up and can be addressed. Doctrinal presentations should not be the primary purpose of in-home visits but doctrines can be discussed if they are brought up by those with whom you are visiting.

> "There are many souls yearning unutterably for light, for assurance and strength beyond what they have been able to grasp. They need to be sought out and labored for patiently, perseveringly. Beseech the Lord in fervent prayer for help. Present Jesus because you know Him as your personal Saviour. Let His melting love, His rich grace, flow forth from human lips. You need not present *doctrinal points* unless questioned. But take the Word, and with tender, yearning love for souls, show them the precious righteousness of Christ, to whom you and they must come to be saved. Welfare Ministry, 92.

The in-home visits allow personal appeals to behavior change, personal appeals to accept Christ as the agent of behavior change in human live.

> "Personal, individual effort and interest for your friends and neighbors will accomplish more than can be estimated. It is for the want of this kind of labor that souls for whom Christ died are perishing.... Your work may accomplish more real good than the more extensive meetings, if they lack in personal effort. When both are combined, with the blessing of God, a more perfect and thorough work may be wrought; but if we can have but one part done, let it be the *individual labor* of opening the Scriptures *in households, making personal appeals,* and talking familiarly with the members of the family, not about things of little importance, but of the great themes of redemption. Let them see that your heart is burdened for the salvation of souls. Welfare Ministry, 93, 94.

Summary

1. Follow-up is important to the success of any health evangelism program.

2. Follow-up programs at the church are poorly attended because a person has been successful and doesn't need to come to the follow-up meeting or a person has failed and is to ashamed to come to a follow-up meeting.

3. Follow-up is best conducted in the home with one-on-one interviews.

4. In home interviews create opportunities for socialization, friendship and Bible Studies.

5. Follow-up creates an opportunity to gather important information that is useful in evaluation of the long term success of your health evangelism program.

13

Evaluating Your Effectiveness

The Importance of Data

We live in a society where business decisions and political strategies are made in response to survey data of some type. Product designs are tested out on focus groups to see what the public might like. The effectiveness of advertising is measured by an increase or decrease in sales. The durability of a product is measured by service records and recalls. The popularity of a product or concept is measured in polls.

All of these activities are methods of evaluation. The effectiveness of any program is demonstrated by some type of evaluation. The church measures the effectiveness of evangelistic efforts by the number of baptisms that occur as a result of the program. Baptisms are the most important measurement the church makes. As previously discussed, there are many steps in the process that leads to baptism and church membership. Baptism is not the best immediate measure of the effectiveness of health evangelism programs.

Standard tools for evaluation of health evangelism are not available off the shelf. As you conduct health evangelism programs in your church you will need to collect and keep track of data. The church has an elaborate mechanism for counting baptisms. It has no process of measuring the effectiveness of health evangelism activities. This is going to be up to you.

Let me illustrate the nature of the problem. When I was the Medical Staff Director of the United States Office on Smoking and Health, the Five-day Plan to Stop Smoking was near it's peak of popularity in the United States and around the world. The U.S. government was interested in preventing people from starting smoking and getting current smokers off cigarettes. We were very interested in the effectiveness of the 5-Day Plan to Stop Smoking.

I traveled the few miles to the Temperance department of the General Conference, then located in Washington, D.C., (in 1980 the Temperance department was joined with the Health Department and is now know as the Health Ministries Department) and conferred with the leaders in charge of the Five-day Plan. I received only two pieces of information. One was that the program had been instrumental in helping 20 million people stop smoking. This statistic was derived from the sales of the Control Booklet which was handed out to each of the program participants.

This statistic is impressive because it is a big number and we like to think that we have helped millions of people. Of course it isn't an accurate number as many organizations stock piled these control booklets to use in future programs. Many of these booklets were eventually used but many were not. The total number of booklets shipped is a very soft number that doesn't reflect an actual count of people served. Hard numbers are needed for convincing statistics.

The second number I received from the Temperance Department of the General Conference was that the effectiveness of the program was very close to 100%. This statistic was derived by counting those who had not had a cigarette during the last 24-hour period of the Five-day Plan to Stop Smoking.

This is a very optimistic number. To be more accurate it would have been better to compare those who were successful on the last night of the program against the number who registered. If 50% of those who registered for the Five-day plan dropped out during the program, you didn't really help those people. They most likely dropped out because they went back to smoking. That would be a 50% success rate even if 100% of those who remained in the program didn't smoke on the last night of the program.

The number of people who quit smoking on the last night of a program is not as important as how many people are still off cigarettes at three months, six months or a year. Later studies have shown that there are very few who relapse and go back to smoking if they successfully stay off cigarettes for a whole year. For this reason, the true, long term, effectiveness of a stop smoking program should be measured at the end of a year and as a denominator should include all who registered for the program.

The Five-day plan, in a very limited way, has been studied in a scientific manner. Sadly, this research was not done by the church and this research was not funded by the church. The church has not used these more accurate numbers in their advertisement of the Five-day Plan and do not usually discuss these numbers in public.

The success rate of the Five-day Plan varies from 10% at the low end up to 35% at the high end at one year. It should be observed that of the "20,000,000" who supposedly have taken the Five-day Plan that less than 1000 have ever been studied in a systematic way. It should also be noted that no other stop smoking program is any more effective than the Five-day Plan.

I have detailed all of this to make an earnest plea for you to design a strong and continuing evaluation component into your health evangelism program. You need truthful, reliable data to prove to yourself, the church and others of the effectiveness of your program. Programs that are shown to produce long term success will receive the blessing of the church and community.

Starting with Paper.

Do not be discouraged by the prospect of having to collect and maintain data. It is not as hard as you think. Start with paper. Everything you can do with a computer you can do with paper. It may take longer but will be just as accurate and reliable.

The kind of data you collect will be essentially the same in every program. I need only discuss the data required only once and it will apply to every program you conduct. You need to collect data at several times during every program.

Data Collection Points in All Programs.

1.   Registration.

2.   During the program.

3.   Last session Questionnaire.

4.   One month follow-up.

5.   Three month follow-up.

6.   Six month follow-up.

7.   One year follow-up

I can make this simple. Much of the same data you collect the first night you will want to collect the last night. This will document what kind of changes have occurred during the program. So, most of the questions asked at registration need to be asked again at the last session.

Each of the follow-up questionnaires should be exactly the same as well. The 1, 3, 6 and 12 month questionnaires are all the same.

Do not be intimidated. Just sit down and write out a few questions. You might want to sit down with other leaders of your program and together develop a list of questions you want to ask. Let me make some suggestions below.

Demographic Data

This is basic information about a person. For every type of health evangelism program you will need this data. I suggest you collect the following.
Demographic Data to Collect.

1. Last Name
2. First Name
3. Middle Name or initial
4. Date of Birth (calculate age from this)
5. Address (You prefer home address)
6. Phone number (get daytime and nighttime phone numbers)
7. Sex (Male or Female)

Optional Demographic Data

8. Marital Status
9. Occupation
10. Number of Children
11. Emergency numbers to call.
12. Religion

First and Last Session Behavioral Data

The data you should collect depends on the nature of your program. If you are going to conduct a stop smoking clinic you should ask questions about smoking. If you are planning a weight management program, you need to ask questions about eating habits. If your are going to conduct an exercise program, you need to ask questions about health and fitness.

The questions you ask should probe a person's knowledge and attitudes about the behavior that needs to be changed. You should ask about a persons health practices. What has a person tried in the past? What do they plan to do at the present? As an example, the following questions are questions I would ask those who registered for a weight control program.

Questions for a weight management program questionnaire.

1.   How much do you weigh today? (Compare with actual weight)

2.   What is the most you have ever weighed?

3.   How many times have you made a serious attempt to lose weight?

4.   How much weight would you like to lose in this 10-week program?

5.   What are foods you snack on the most? List three.

6.   What is the most weight you have lost following a diet?

7.   How many others in your immediate family would you say are overweight?

8.   Do you believe that God helps a person lose weight?

9.   At what age would you say that you were first overweight?

10. Do you have high cholesterol?

11. Do you have diabetes?

12. Do you have high blood pressure?

13. Has your doctor advised you to lose weight for health reasons?

14. Do you have a regular exercise program?

You can add or subtract questions from this list. Don't make the questionnaire too long. It shouldn't take more than 5-10 minutes to complete. You don't want a bottle neck to develop in the registration area.

You should ask many of the same questions on the last session. By comparing answers from the last session with the answers given at registration, you can document changes in attitude, beliefs and practices. If a smoker said that he or she didn't believe that God helped smokers quit on the first night but on the last night had changed their mind and now did believe that God helps smokers quit you can see that this person is closer to the kingdom.

Data Collection During the Program

For a weight control program you will want to have people weigh in privately at each session. There should be data collected each week of the program to document behavior change on an on going basis. I like to use a "Progress Card." This card is given out every session of the program and then collected when a participant returns the next week. New cards are distributed again when last weeks cards are picked up.

The person trying to lose weight should keep score of several behaviors daily throughout each week. The data collected should be identical from week to week. I like to document the following data in a weight loss program.

Progress Card Data collected for each day of the week.

1. Amount eaten at each meal.

   (Same as usual, less than usual, much less than usual or more than usual)

2. Frequency of between meal snacks.

3. Frequency and duration of exercise each day.

4. Avoidance of specific food items selected by the participant.

5. Daily prayer for help with dieting.

6. Contacting partners for encouragement

Another type of data you can collect is to document the involvement of the church members who are volunteers in your health evangelism program. The purpose of the gospel is to make and keep church members active in God's service. Involvement with health evangelism programs qualifies as the highest type of service and it honors God. So, count how many volunteers you have and how often they help.

Keep track of the number of church members who attend every preparatory meeting, those who help with each session, those who are involved in follow-up and those who are involved at all levels. These data about those who conduct the health evangelism program gives you an index of activity for your local church.

The effectiveness of your program depends not only on the number of community members who attend and whose lives are changed but also on the number of church members who are involved and whose lives are changed by service.

Designate one or more persons to collect and hold the data you generate for later analysis. Be diligent in data collection and in analysis. This will be the proof of the effectiveness of your program. The numbers you can point to will justify your program to your church board and also to church administrators at other levels as well. You data will also be useful in justifying your program to your community at large. Numbers will be useful in future advertising. You may want to present your results at a ministerial retreat or even write an article about your health evangelism program.

Data Analysis

Data analysis is a scary concept for many. There are professionals whose lives are dedicated to data analysis and you might not have any of these specialists in your church. Do not fear. If you collect the data you can figure out what to do with it.

Data analysis starts with questions. The data has been collected and sits before you. Ask some questions.

One question is, "How many people attended our program?"

You can answer that question by counting how many people registered for the program. That is easy enough. But, if you stop to think about it, the attendance each night of the program varied some what. In most programs attendance falls during the program. How will you account for that? I compensate for the variation by counting "person-visits." Count everyone every time they step through the door. This is how it works. If you had ten people register for a five-session program and everyone came to every session you would have 10 X 5 = 50 person-visits. If your attendance at each session was: 10, 8, 5, 9 and 7, you would just add this up. The answer is 39 person-visits to your program. This number would be the same if you had one person attend 39 sessions or 39 people attend a one session program. It would result in 39 person-visits.

You might want to know how many people attended all five sessions, how many attended four, how many attended three sessions etc. You have the data and can extract the numbers. You might want to know how many men and how many women attended your program. You might want to know what ages attended your program. This would tell you if your program was attractive to an older or younger crowd. Go to your registration forms and make a list.

Most importantly, how many people changed their behavior as a result of the program. You know what the initial behavior pattern was by documenting what the group was doing the night they registered. You know what changes occurred during the program by documenting the behavior changes on the last night of the program. You will document the long term success of your program by counting up what people are doing at one month, three months, six months and a year.

You should use the number of people who registered at the beginning of the program as your denominator. This will result in the lowest success rate but is a more accurate measure of your overall success. Some will want to use the number of people who completed the program as the denominator. It is not wrong to do it either way. It is just important to disclose which method you used to calculate your success rate.

Let's illustrate this principle. Lets say that 10 people signed up for a stop smoking program and five actually finished the program. On the last night all five had stopped smoking. At a year three were still off cigarettes. How could you analyze this? At the last night all who attended the last night were off cigarettes, so, by that measure you had a 100% success rate. If you use those who registered as the denominator your success rate is only 50%. At a year, if you use the last night attendance your success rate at a year is 60% but if you use the more conservative registration figure of 10 your one year success rate is only 30%. It doesn't matter which way you calculate your success rate just so you disclose the numbers you used and how you calculated your success rate.

It will be important to document how many community members who are not members of your church attended your program. If all who attended the hypothetical program referred to above were not members of your church, you could share with the pastor, church members, and church administrators at various levels, that you had 39 person-visits by nonmembers of your church.

Having nonmembers attend your church are important steps that will lead to baptisms at some time in the future. You are demonstrating that your program brings nonmembers to the church.

Let's look at this another way. Count every session where there was contact and interaction between church members and non-church members. If a church member led a small group, there would be a member-to-nonmember contact. You could say that not only was there a 39 person-visits to the church to report, but that there were 39 member to nonmember personal contacts generated by your program as well. If there was at least one phone call to all 10 registrants every day for all five days, you have 50 more member to nonmember contacts being made to swell the total to 89 member to nonmember contacts. (50 by telephone and 39 in person.)

Further, if there were three follow-up visits to the five who finished your program during the year following the program that will generate another 15 member to nonmember contacts bringing the total for the year to 104 member to nonmember contacts for your program that lasted five nights.

There will probably be a couple of Bible studies started as a result of this program. There will be several church members involved in activities who were just inactive, bench warming Christians before they became involved in your health evangelism program. You can demonstrate that your health evangelism activity is waking up formerly inactive members.

Generate data, keep data, analyze data, share data, publish data. In this way your program will demonstrate its value and will attract additional resources and will spread far and wide.

Computer Analysis

It is not necessary to have a computer to do all I have discussed above. However, all the data analysis I discussed above can be done more quickly and easily on a computer. The data can be entered into a database program and the analysis can be done whenever you want to do it. Your registration data goes into the computer as well as the progress cards during the program. Your last session questionnaire and all follow-up questionnaires are entered. Then you sit down and do an analysis of your data.

To do this on a computer, you will need a database program and someone who can configure the program to match your various questionnaires. The same computer person can help with data analysis. Data base programs I have used include, dBASE, Microsoft Access, and Alpha Five. There are several other fine database programs that would serve your purposes just as well.

If there is anyone in your church who operates small computers, invite them to your planning meetings and see if they can help you put your health evangelism program on the computer. It would be best if the data could be entered as you go along.

I have had data entry persons enter data each night during the program as we were conducting it. They would print results immediately. At the end of each program I would be able to share with the group various statistics showing how well the group did during the previous week. For a weight control program we would identify the person who had lost the most weight so far. Who lost the most weight in the past week etc. Those who were doing particularly well were given some recognition. We did this for the males and females. Data entry and quick analysis allowed us to provide up-to-the-minute statistics. This was appreciated by those who attended. They knew we had our finger on the pulse of the program.

Another way to collect, enter and analyze data is to utilize a "web server." In this way the data from many separate programs can be kept at a central location. Aggregate data could quickly prove the effectiveness of a new health evangelism program. Individuals with computer access could register their progress with a "monitoring/accountability" program they can access on the web.

Publish Your Data

In the scientific community, publishing data in peer reviewed journals is an important activity. For health evangelism, presentations and publications are just as important. Health evangelism will never rise to the importance it deserves until its effectiveness is demonstrated. This requires careful data collection and analysis but also requires publicizing your results.

It is not necessary to publish your findings in a scientific journal. Publish your findings in your church news letter. Present your data to the church as a whole during a Sabbath service. See if you can report on your success at various ministerial meetings and retreats. Share your information with other churches and at camp meeting. Call a special meeting of churches in your geographical area to be held at your church where you can present concepts of health evangelism and share the results of your efforts.

The early SDA church grew and remained cohesive in large measure due to the publishing work. Health evangelism will grow strong as its effectiveness is proclaimed and published abroad.

Summary

1. Data collection is important. It validates the effectiveness of health evangelism.

2. Collect demographic data regarding age, sex, race and other characteristics.

3.   Questionnaires administered the first and then the last night of the program will document what behavior changes have occurred immediately during the health evangelism program.

4.   Data collected periodically during a year of follow-up will document the long term success of your health evangelism program.

5.   Analysis of your data is quite simple. Ask questions and then tabulate the data to provide answers. Computer analysis is quicker but not necessary to get results.

6.   Publish your results once you have enough information that will be of interest to others. Church papers at state and national levels will help promote health evangelism.

14

Networking and Marketing your Programs

Networking is the process of exchanging ideas, data, and even program participants with other agencies, programs and churches. Your health evangelism program will generate ideas and data. This information needs to be communicated. You need to communicate with your own home church. Your church members need to be moved into action. They can join and help your program succeed or they can form other health evangelism programs to serve the needs of your community.

Communicate with church administrators at all levels. You should attend meetings to share your success and you will want to publish your findings in appropriate journals. With all of this networking, don't forget to interface with the community as well. Service organizations and various governmental agencies need to know what you are doing. Local, state, and federal organizations may be interested in your health evangelism programs. Voluntary organizations such as the Heart Association, Lung Association, Cancer Society and Diabetes Association should know what you are doing in your health evangelism programs.

Once you have some good data to share, make the rounds and share your success. This will result in the fruits of networking which is referrals into your program from other programs in your community.

Let's take smoking cessation as an example. The Cancer Society, Lung Association and Heart Association, each encourages people to stop smoking. These organizations occasionally conduct smoking cessation programs. These organizations have films, literature and displays that discourage smoking.

When you network with these organizations you create an opportunity to use the excellent materials they have developed. Using good material from other organizations helps legitimize your operations and shows a spirit of cooperation with outside agencies.

You may be invited to join one of these voluntary organizations and participate in their activities. This is a good idea. I have served at various levels as a volunteer with the American Cancer Society, American Heart Association, and the
Texas Interagency Counsel on Smoking and Health. This was profitable for my
health evangelism activities as it gave me access to great materials I could use in
my own programs and enhanced my credibility with my audience.

This is a two-way street. If you were to use some of the materials from the
American Cancer Society in a smoking cessation program, they would want to
know how many people attended and how much literature you distributed. The
Cancer Society is anxious to document the effectiveness of their own programs
and your use of their material makes them more successful as well.

This is more than advertising. You are developing relationships with community organizations. As your effectiveness and reputation grows, community agencies will be proud to affiliate with you and will refer individuals to you health
evangelism program for the services you provide.

So, reach outward. Find organizations with similar goals. Use materials that
have been developed by others when it is consistent with your own message.
Receive program participants by referral from other organizations.

Referral

There will be many individuals who will attend your health evangelism program
who will need more help than your program can provide. It is important to establish a roster of organizations to whom you can refer problem participants.

The clinically sick need the care of a medical professional. It is your function
to change behaviors but not to treat active disease processes. Those who are ill
need to be under the care of a physician in the local health care system. If a person doesn't have a doctor, you should know how to find a doctor for a person
who needs one.

Those who are offended by the spiritual content of your health evangelism
program need a secular program to attend that omits the spiritual emphasis. You
should catalog the various behavior change programs in your region that address
the problems your participants have, just in case they become upset with you and
need a referral.

Then there will be those who simply fail to change their behaviors. These people may be successful for a short period of time but fail in the long run. You have
done all you can. Your church members have prayed for them and called them
but they still fail. Such individuals need to be removed from their day to day

environment and referred to a live-in program for more intensive behavior modification. Several better living centers are listed on page 22.

These organizations take people for 7-28 days and control their diet, environment, sleep and exercise. A person who has had trouble changing behavior at home is more likely to succeed in an institutional setting. These centers are relatively expensive to attend. Insurance programs usually don't cover the costs of behavior change programs. If there is a person from your church who would benefit from such a program and doesn't have sufficient resources to attend, perhaps your church or someone in your church could help pay the expenses.

These Better Living Centers have operated as autonomous, self-supporting organizations for decades. They advertise widely to receive their clients. Clients come from their homes, take the program and then return home without any personalized follow-up. Not so with clients you refer to better living centers.

A problem participant from your church who attends a live-in program at a better living center will have friends back in the "home" church who know them and who have tried to help them and who are praying for them. As soon as the live-in program is completed, these participants will be returning to your community. You can help them maintain their new behaviors.

Don't Compromise

Your health evangelism program should be a spiritual program. Do not apologize for this and do not make compromises with anyone to make yourself more acceptable or more attractive to the secular or governmental agencies with whom you network.

There was a time when I advised a local pastor who was wanting to run a Five-day Plan to Stop Smoking in his church to contact the American Cancer Society to obtain a couple of films and some literature I recommended.

This pastor called me back a day or two later and was disappointed because the American Cancer Society would not share any of their materials with him. The reason was because he charged a nominal fee for his program and they didn't want their "free" material to be "sold." This of course was a misunderstanding and misinterpretation of the facts by the American Cancer Society.

I contacted the Cancer Society and explained the situation to them and told them of my background in the field of smoking and health. As a result of my phone call the Cancer Society delivered the films and brochures requested by the pastor to his door and I was invited to become a member of the Help Smokers

Quit committee for the local chapter of the Cancer Society. In a few weeks I was invited to sit on the board of directors for the Cancer Society.

During a phone call, taking my food order for my first board of directors meeting, I was offered a roast beef sandwich which was going to be delivered to the boardroom from a local fast food restaurant. I declined stating that I was a vegetarian and would just grab a bite at the hospital before I came. They volunteered that the restaurant also had a beautiful chief's salad if I wanted that.

Well, I was early to my very first board meeting and recognized my place at the table because there was one big salad and thirteen roast beef sandwiches placed around the table. As board members came in almost everyone asked, "Who is this and how did he get a salad?" I explained that I was a vegetarian, Seventh-day Adventist and was a new board member.

Of course, beef is a clean meat, and eating a beef sandwich once a month at a board meeting is a minimal compromise of my standards and no one would think less of me for eating a beef sandwich. It would be a compromise over a little thing however, and I chose not to compromise.

Board members were delighted to know that there were other options on the menu other than the traditional roast beef sandwich. At a subsequent board meeting, several months later, I was pleased to see 12 salads and only one roast beef sandwich. The person who ate the beef sandwich apologized for not wanting to eat the "rabbit food" the rest of us were eating. He was a beef man and wasn't going to change. We were all forgiving of him.

The point is, do not compromise your standards or your health evangelism program in the process of networking. There will be many points at which you will have an opportunity to compromise. Don't do it. Others will always want you to eliminate the spiritual emphasis in your program. Don't do it. There are plenty of Godless programs people can go to. Your programs are designed to be evangelistic. Your health evangelism activities involve the church, church members and the gospel.

I ran across an outstanding example of compromise when I was promoting the Breathe Free Plan to Stop Smoking in Europe at the time when I was connected with the Health and Temperance Department of the General Conference of Seventh-day Adventists. I was trying to get people to try the new Breathe Free Plan in place of the older Five-day Plan to Stop Smoking. I was also trying to get people to use their local churches as program locations. I stressed the importance of using church members as helpers in conducting the Breathe Free Program.

In certain European countries the older Five-day Plan to Stop Smoking was given official recognition by the government. Those who conducted the Five-day

Plan to Stop Smoking were paid by the government to conduct these programs for the public. The Five-day Plan was being presented without a spiritual component. It was conducted in public places—not churches. And it was conducted by health professionals—without the added benefit that would have come from the services of volunteer church members. This is a sad example of networking that resulted in a compromise of the basic principles of health evangelism. In my opinion this weakened the Five-day Plan to the point where it became relatively useless to the church.

In my opinion, the Seventh-day Adventist church doesn't need to be conducting health education programs that are totally secular. To do so represents a serious compromise of the principles of health evangelism which are put forth in this book. Networking is important but not if you have to compromise what you are doing. Oh, yes, compromise is a fine thing under many circumstances but not if it results in a diversion from the fundamentals of health evangelism.

Advertising

Health evangelism programs need advertising and promotion to get started. It has been my experience that as soon as a program becomes well established in the community almost all advertising can be decreased. Usually, by the third or fourth program you will be so well known that further use of advertising will not be needed.

It is important to have brochures that describe your health evangelism program. You should schedule future programs 12 months in advance. It is good to lay plans for a year at a time. You brochures should have this schedule printed in it. At the end of each health evangelism program your audience wants to know when the next program is going to be held. Give each participant a quantity of brochures for them to hand out to their friends and neighbors. Most of your new participants will come from word of mouth promotion by previous participants.

A good source of referrals is from health professionals. The health professionals in your church should have a supply of brochures for their office. They can refer their patients who need specific behaviors changed. A referral from a health professional is more likely to result in a person coming than from any other source.

Don't limit your contact to just health professionals who are members of your church. Deliver a supply of brochures to all of the doctors, and other practitioners in your community. Family practitioners, internal medicine doctors, pulmonary specialists, cardiologists, and cancer specialists will all be glad to refer their patients to your church for behavior change classes.

Other media can be useful. Regional papers will often run a feature story about your health evangelism program, especially if you purchase some advertising space. Radio and TV have community calendars where special events like your health evangelism program can receive attention.

About one to two weeks before a new health evangelism program starts I like to send a letter to all previous participants to remind them that a new program is about to begin. Backsliders can come back and recycle themselves if they have slipped or perhaps they have family or friends to whom they would like to recommend your program. A large number of new participants come from a personal letter like this.

I also promote each program to all who have attended any program of any type at the church. It keeps your calendar fresh in their mind and past participants from one program might be interested in some other program you conduct.

Posters are useful when put up in local business and professional offices. Posters look best if done professionally but do the best you can with the talent and resources you have in your church.

Summary

1. As a health evangelism program becomes effective in helping people change it will also become popular in the community. This creates opportunities for networking.

2. Refer people to other programs in the community if you are not able to take care of a person's needs.

3. Promote your health evangelism activities to other community agencies so they can refer people to your program.

4. In developing connections with other agencies don't compromise the essential elements of your health evangelism programs. Compromise results in increased popularity and acceptance but limits the soul-winning potential of your programs.

5. Advertizing on radio, in print, in church bulletins and in direct mail outs are all methods that can be used to get your health evangelism program well

attended. It is usually the case that advertizing isn't needed once a program is well established. There will be a waiting list for upcoming programs.

15

How to Deal with Special Issues

Health evangelism activities in the church will sometimes result in special problems that will cripple your effectiveness. These problems and issues will come up repeatedly. How you approach these problems is up to you and your staff. You need to be aware of them. I will review the ways I have dealt with these problems, but you may need to try a different solution depending on your circumstances.

Independence

What should be the relationship of your health evangelism program to your local church, the local conference or union conference? Well, to begin with, it is unlikely that your church or church administration is doing anything in the way of health evangelism, so your program will be totally independent as it begins.

As your health evangelism program becomes increasingly successful there will be attempts by others to assume control or management of your program. This will be true if your health evangelism program attracts wide interest among non-church members in the community and baptisms eventually result. This will be especially true if your health evangelism program makes considerable amounts of money as a result of fees collected or investment by interested parties.

I believe that successful health evangelism programs will spread to many other churches. As this occurs, it is only natural for church administrators to want to have some involvement or control of your program. What should be done?

There should be no secrecy or covert activity. Your committees, your data and your financial records should be open for any responsible individual or organization to inspect. You should be open with your church and church administrators who show an interest in your program.

You should cooperate with churches and church administrators. The blessing and endorsement of local churches and church administrators will go a long way to legitimize your work and will open doors of access to other churches in many places.

Cooperation however, doesn't imply control. Pray for wisdom on how to approach this problem. Relinquish management and promotion of your health evangelism program only if it appears that it is the best step for God's work.

A successful health evangelism program is not an opportunity for you to become famous or rich. Successful health evangelism advances God's work. The whole process should be controlled by God and your role may need to diminish so the church and God's work can get the credit for the success of health evangelism.

On the other hand, God may need you to keep a steady hand on the health evangelism programs you have developed. You may need to stay connected with your programs in order to preserve them. God will guide. Don't be selfish when success comes.

Copyright

Any materials you develop should be copyrighted in your name. This is not to guarantee recognition or profit for you, but to protect your material from being stolen and misappropriated by others who may not understand health evangelism as you do. I have known people who developed useful materials but left their product in the public domain only to have it stolen by someone else who copyrighted that material. Those who copyrighted the stolen material then turned around and prohibited the original developer of the material from promoting or using their own material. What a sad lesson.

Your goal should be to see health evangelism spread far and wide. Copyright the materials you develop and then generously allow others to use them. Do not copyright materials to restrict health evangelism or to make a profit, although making a living from the work you do is appropriate. Do not use health evangelism programs as a venue to promote, distribute or sell health supplements, special foods, vitamins or minerals.

Commercialism

Some individual health evangelism programs may become commercially successful. If you are an employee of the church at some level of administration, I would expect that you shouldn't make any profit from a health evangelism program you develop. The church is paying your salary and providing you with benefits. Any product you develop while working for the church ought to be the property of the church organization.

The situation is different if you earn a living for yourself. If a health evangelism program you develop and copyright becomes a commercial success you will have to be careful in the choices you make. It is appropriate for you to make a living wage. Profits from any health evangelism program however, should largely be used to advance health evangelism among local churches. The local church that uses your program should realize enough profit to offset all expenses and provide that church with enough margin to promote other health evangelism activities in that local church and the surrounding community.

Dictatorial Leadership

When a health evangelism program becomes successful there is a human tendency for the developer to become proud. There is a tendency to think that the success of a program is largely due to your personal charisma, talent and skill. There follows a dictatorial, controlling environment that hampers success.

It is best to develop and promote programs with a committee. God blesses us when we work together to advance His cause. Making moves from the consensus developed when a group of workers have shared, studied, and prayed with one another is superior to dictatorial decisions. This is always true.

Health Fanatics

Health evangelism is given a bad name and is discredited by health fanatics. Where do health fanatics come from? The devil has cleverly claimed the extremes of health. There are the couch potatoes who eat Pizza, drink beer and munch on chips whose blob like bodies drape over their sofa for hours each weekend. Then there are the health fanatics who have no (or only a limited) education in health matters. These people have come to believe one or more of a hundred bogus health theories that abound in our culture.

These fanatics go to extremes in drink and diet. Many are devout church members who think their actions are condoned by Scripture or Spirit of Prophecy. These fanatics will be quick to volunteer to help you with your health evangelism program. They will often want an opportunity to present their ideas or products in their small group or at a regular session. Kindly, but firmly avoid these people. They will only confuse your audience and will taint your good reputation.

Spiritual Zealots

These are devout church members. They have a zeal for God that can be useful but may need to be tempered, especially in the early phases of a health evangelism program. The gospel presented in your health evangelism program should be problem-specific and free from religious jargon or distinctive doctrines.

These spiritually zealous individuals will want to help with your health evangelism program. If not instructed carefully they may use your health program as an opportunity to preach to your participants. They will not confine their spiritual conversation to the health problems at hand. They will rush to doctrinal topics and will use their small groups to discuss the distinctive doctrines of the church. They don't bring just the milk of the word but meat as well.

Don't necessarily give up on this group. They do want to help but they bring too much with them. If they can be convinced to go slow and to confine a discussion of God's help to the behavioral problem at hand they can be useful.

Spiritual Novices

These church members set a bad example. They don't believe in the health message. They don't practice the health message. When someone who wants to live a healthier life gets to know one of these people they will become discouraged. These people often talk a lot of the love of God and how he saves to the uttermost. They want you to, "Only, believe." How you live is secondary to trust in God.

These church members, when it comes right down to it, think that most health evangelism is a form of salvation by works. They abuse their Christian liberty by living degenerate lives in various ways. These church members often wake up when they develop diabetes or have a heart attack or a stroke. These members are then willing to help. Don't give up on these members. If you have an obese church member who wants to help in a weight control program you can do one of two things. You can request that they take the program along with public members to demonstrate that they are serious about weight control. Once these church members have developed a measure of control over their habits and have a new or deeper relationship with God, they are ready to be a helper in the next program.

Or, you can take a chance and plug them into your program. I have used massively obese church members as partners in small groups. These people were always the ones to lose the most weight. They were making painful application to their own lives at each step of the way just like others in the groups. Their lives were literally on the line. Most did well. Those who didn't do well usually didn't want to help in the next program.

Nutritional Supplements

The nutritional supplement business is a multibillion dollar industry in the United States. In every church I have visited or been a member there are people who are distributors of some special formulation of vitamins or minerals or herbal products. In a word, avoid this whole area.

It is especially distressing to me when I see pastors and their wives promoting these products in their congregation and community. Many of these people feel that the use of these nutritional pills or potions will help keep you off "drug" medication and are consistent with the writings of Ellen White. This is not the case as clearly made by Dr. Mervyn G. Hardinge's book, *A Physician Explains Ellen White's Counsel on Drugs, Herbs, & Natural Remedies* published by the Review and Herald Publishing Association. (2001)

Do not advocate or promote the use of any nutritionally or vitamin supplements in any health evangelism program. God made food. Man extracts small components of plants and promotes them as being better than the original. Food is wonderful. Food is adequate. Stick with good foods and forget the pills.

Cures For Disease

Those who are sick are looking for a cure. Let the sick go to doctors and hospitals. Health evangelism is about prevention not about cures. Living right may make your diabetes, weight and blood pressure improve. Exercise may reduce your risk of a heart attack.

Your health evangelism program should be about preventing disease by controlling harmful behaviors NOT curing people of their diseases. You should not be in the business of practicing medicine without a license. Do not promise to cure anything. You can prevent or reduce the risk of cancer, you can prevent or reduce the risk of a stroke or heart attack but you cannot cure cancer or cure a stroke or cure a heart attack. The modern medical system works on those who have become sick. This is the work for hospitals and doctors in your community. You must not try to do their work for them.

Hospitals and doctors spend little or no time on prevention. Prevention requires behavior change which is so difficult and usually impossible without God's help. Stick to behavior change issues and stay away from cures.

Food Demonstrations

Food demonstrations present special problems. In order for everyone to see clearly, an overhead mirror or some type of closed circuit TV will be required. If the group is small then all participants can crowd around a table.

If you are going to serve samples of various dishes that are being demonstrated, this should be done in proximity to a regular meal so as to not be eating between meals. Food served as part of a food demonstration may substitute for a meal if sufficient samples are served to constitute a good meal.

Measure out all ingredients so that the recipe can be put together rapidly. If baking or prolonged cooking is required, have a batch completed and ready to serve so there won't be additional delay in cooking food.

Recipes are important. Ideally, they should be low in saturated fat and cholesterol and should have limited sugar content. We should only demonstrate recipes that represent good nutrition. Recipes must pass the "taste test." The food should look good and taste good as well!

Those demonstrating a recipe should be familiar with the recipe they are presenting. I don't mean just having fixed it a few times at home to get used to the recipe, but it should be a recipe that has been in regular use by the presenter at home for years.

Church members are usually so truthful that if they don't eat the food they are demonstrating at home on a regular basis they will confess that they have been trying all week to get the recipe just right. I have been asked if a certain concoction looked OK right in the middle of a demonstration. These small errors suggest that members of your church don't eat this food and are unfamiliar with it.

I had a sweet little old Italian lady in one program demonstrate a soup recipe that had been in her family for generations. She had learned the recipe from her mother. It had a couple of "secret" ingredients that made the soup "special." This lady with her strong accent just won the audience over. Everyone loved her soup. Everyone took the recipe home. The evening was a great success.

Yes, you should screen recipes to see that they are appropriate from a nutritional point of view but it is so important to be authentic that I would rather use family recipes that are in constant use rather than some recipe a nutritionist hands out for you to try.

Summary

1. Independence can be bad. Cooperate with others but don't let others run, control or take over a program you have developed.

2. Copyright all original materials.

3. Don't be dictatorial.

4. Avoid health fanatics and untested ideas and cures.

5. Avoid spiritual fanatics.

6. Put spiritual novices to work but watch them carefully as they can drift.

7. Nutritional supplements are big business but are not to be part of health evangelism.

8. Health evangelism is for changing behavior and preventing disease. Refer the sick to other resources. Do not treat the sick in a church based health evangelism program.

9. Make all demonstrations utilizing local talent. Avoid complicated presentations by people who don't live or eat that way.

Appendix

1. Sample article for church newsletter about a weight control program.

The heat of summer makes us long for fall and cooler weather. Fall is also when we start up Best Weigh again. This year Best Weigh starts on Tuesday, September 9, 2003 and runs through November 11.

Best Weigh is a unique form of witnessing to the community. It is based on the concept that behavior change is possible—especially with God's help. Losing weight is a lot harder than controlling most other addictions. You can give up tobacco, alcohol and drugs but you must continue to eat. Constant vigilance is needed to control the appetite. With Best Weigh you learn to depend on God daily for strength to fight temptation.

Best Weigh is a really good program to offer the community because many of our members need it as much as our neighbors do. This keeps us from having a superiority complex. For instance we used to relish doing smoking cessation programs because none of us smoked. We secretly and sometimes openly gloated over the fact that we had overcome on that particular point. When we do Best Weigh it keeps us humble because it is obvious we need weight control and God's help as much as anyone.

Best Weigh provides an opportunity to get to know our Christian neighbors in a context that is non-threatening to us. They come to our church to learn the principles of Best Weigh. There are witnessing programs that require us to go and meet people in their own homes or in some public place. This makes many of us uncomfortable. If you want to witness in a most comfortable setting get involved with Best Weigh.

Best Weigh is the effort of many people. There are some who are up front a lot giving lectures. Others, who are just as important, work as group leaders, facilitating conversation at the tables where we meet in small groups.

There will be four meetings to help get the Best Weigh organized for the fall. Please volunteer to help in the fall Best Weigh. Our first organizational meeting will be on August 12. These will be in the fellowship hall at 7:00pm. Please get involved in this church project.

Sincerely,

Elvin Adams, MD
Director of Best Weigh

2. Second sample article for church newsletter regarding a weight control program.

It's Best Weigh Time Again.

We do Best Weigh twice a year, once in the spring and once in the fall. Best Weigh is a weight management program, but it is much more.

Best Weigh teaches you how to eat right. We encourage a vegetarian diet, which has been shown to reduce cholesterol levels and result in fewer heart attacks and strokes. The vegetarian diet also reduces your risk of cancer. Learn about the advantages of a vegetarian diet at Best Weigh.

Best Weigh brings friends from other faiths to our church. This gives you a chance to get to know your neighbors in a comfortable setting. Best Weigh gives you a non-threatening way to be a Christian witness and counselor.

If you haven't had blood work recently, Best Weigh give you a chance to have a chemistry profile for free. Helpers get before and after laboratory studies including triglycerides and both good and bad cholesterol levels without cost.

Best Weigh doesn't touch on any of the distinctive doctrines of the SDA church but we provide a health promoting service for the community and make new friends. It is a lot of fun and there is room for many kinds of helpers.

Our next Best Weigh starts on Tuesday, February 25 and runs every Tuesday evening from 7:00 to 8:30 p.m. through April 29. If you need to attend Best Weigh to shed a few holiday pounds put this on your calender now.

There will be four organizing meetings for Best Weigh beginning on January 28, 2003. If you want to help out in Best Weigh in some way please attend each of these meetings.

Sincerely,

Elvin Adams, MD
Director of Best Weigh

3. Sample church bulletin announcement for a weight control program.

Fall Best Weigh starts September 9 and runs through November 11. Plan on attending with a friend who needs to lose weight. We need volunteers who will help with Best Weigh. Our organizing meetings will start on August 4 in the fellowship hall at 7:00pm. Come help make this fall Best Weigh the best we have ever done.

4. Sample letter to past participants about a scheduled weight control program.

BEST WEIGH

Burleson S.D.A. Church
601 South Burleson Boulevard
Burleson, TX 76028

Phone(817) 295-7141

August 20, 2003

Dear Friends:

The fall Best Weigh program is just around the corner. It starts at 7:00 p.m. on Tuesday September 7, 2004 in the fellowship hall of the Burleson SDA Church. Best Weigh will run each Thursday night for 10 weeks ending on November 9, 2004.

If you, your family, friends, or neighbors want to attend please call and register with the church secretary at 295-7141. Many will lose 10-20 lbs. Some will lose 30. Many have been successful in keeping it off over the summer.

The pricing is flexible to meet your needs.

Best Weigh for one person

With blood work at the beginning and end.	$45
With no blood work.	$30

Best Weigh for a family (up to 4 in the same household)

With blood work at the beginning and end.	$60
With no blood work.	$40
Blood work for each family member who wants it.	$15

I am excited. Make plans now to attend Best Weigh. Shed those pounds before the holidays. Learn to keep those unwanted pounds off.

Sincerely,

Elvin Adams, M.D., M.P.H.
Director of Best Weigh

5. Letter to health professionals asking for referrals to a weight control program.

Best Weigh
Burleson S.D.A. Church
601 South Burleson Boulevard
Burleson, TX 76028

Phone(817) 295-7141

August 20, 2003

Dear Doctor:

We are pleased to announce the fall BEST WEIGH program will begin Thursday, September 9 and will run 10 weeks through November 11. This is a very sensible weight loss program based on eating less and exercising more. We do a chemistry profile with cholesterol, triglycerides, HDL and LDL at the beginning and the end.

All meetings are in the Living Resource Center (fellowship hall) of the Burleson S.D.A. church and begin at 7:00pm. The total fee (including all lab work) is $45. All participants receive a workbook. They are weighed weekly. Many will lose 10-20 lbs during the program. A few will lose 30 pounds.

Would you encourage your patients who need to lose weight to attend? Enclosed are a few handouts. The lectures are given by medical doctors and nutritionists.

I thank you and your patients will thank you.

Sincerely,

Elvin E. Adams, M.D., M.P.H.
Director of Best Weigh

6. Master list of volunteers for the various jobs at a weight control program.

Group Partners

      Group 1   _____

                        _____

      Group 2   _____

                        _____

      Group 3   _____

                        _____

Group 4   _____
            _____

Group 5   _____
            _____

Group 6   _____
            _____

Group 7   _____
            _____

Group 8   _____
            _____

Group 10   _____
            _____

Master of Ceremonies   _____

Lecturers   _____
                              _____
                              _____

Spiritual Topics & Slimming Behaviors   _____
                              _____

Registration   _____
                              _____
                              _____
                              _____

Greeters   _____
                              _____
                              _____
                              _____

Audio   _____
                              _____

Set Up Overhead Projector & Screen _____

Weigh In _____

_____

_____

_____

Set Up & Take Down Chairs and Tables _____

_____

_____

_____

Get and Present Prizes _____

Data Entry _____

_____

Materials Duplication and Collation _____

_____

Materials Distribution each Session _____

_____

Table Demonstration of Lecture _____

_____

7. Sample program elements and duration of events for a weight control program.

CLASS 1

Greeting

Registration

Blood Draw

Weigh In

Welcome (When majority in)   5 min

Fundamentals of Best Weigh	30 min
Spiritual Resources	10 min
Groups	30 min

CLASS 2

Greeting

Late registration

Weigh In

Welcome at 7:00

Laboratory Results	10 min
Exercise Lecture	20 min
Spiritual Resources &Slimming Behaviors	10 min
Recognition and Prizes	5 min
Groups	30 min

CLASS 3-10

Weigh In

Welcome at 7:00

Main Lecture: Nutrition, Exercise, Best Weigh	25 min
Spiritual Resources &Slimming Behaviors	10 min
Recognition and Prizes	5 min
Groups	30 min

CLASS 9

Blood Draw

CLASS 10
Distribute Lab Results
Discuss Lab Results

8. Individual Weight Loss Graphic.

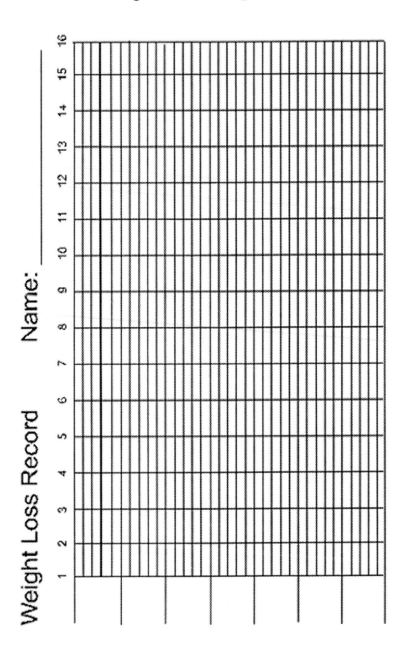

9. Sample individual weight loss record

The Individual Weight Loss Record on the previous page is designed to be very flexible so that everyone can use it no matter how much they weigh or how little they weigh. The left hand side is marked off in 5 pound divisions for the major lines and one pound divisions for the smallest lines.

At the first session, a persons weight is entered by placing a dot on the left margin of the graph near the top. The scale would then be filled in with pounds decreasing to the bottom of the page. This is best illustrated with an example. Let's say someone weighed in at 322 pounds. You would designate the top mark on the upper left hand corner as 325 pounds. The next big line down would become 320 pounds and then next big line down the left side would be 320 pounds and so on until you reached the bottom of the page. In this case the bottom most big line on the left side of the page would be 275 pounds.

The dot indicating this week's weight would be placed on the line that is 3 lines down from the top 325 pound mark. (This of course would be two small lines above the 320 line mark). Every one customizes their own weight loss record so that their beginning weight is somewhere close to the top of the left hand side of the page. If participants are inclined to compare records with one another everyone's graph will essentially look alike as they will have all started in the upper left hand corner of the graph.

When participants weigh in at the end of the first week a dot is entered along the vertical 1 line. After two weeks the weight is entered on the 2 line and so on. If your program is 10 sessions long the last night's weight will be recorded on the 9 line. There is room for a participant to continue recording their progress at home in the weeks that follow the program.

10. BMI. Body Mass Index.

On the next page is a table used to calculate BMI. All scientific weight programs use the BMI to measure obesity. A BMI of 20-25 is normal for men and women regardless of their height or bone structure. A BMI of 26-30 is in the overweight category. A BMI of 30 or above is considered obese.

BMI	25	26	27	28	29	30	31	32	33	34	35	36	37	38	39	40
4'10"	119	124	129	134	138	143	148	153	158	162	167	172	177	181	186	191
4'11"	124	128	133	138	143	148	153	158	163	168	173	178	183	188	193	198
5'0"	128	133	138	143	148	153	158	164	169	174	179	184	189	194	199	204
5'1"	132	137	143	148	153	158	164	169	174	180	185	190	195	201	206	211
5'2"	136	142	147	153	158	164	169	175	180	186	191	196	202	207	213	218
5'3"	141	146	152	158	163	169	175	180	186	192	197	203	208	214	220	225
5'4"	145	151	157	163	169	174	180	186	192	198	203	209	215	221	227	233
5'5"	150	156	162	168	174	180	186	192	198	204	210	216	222	228	234	240
5'6"	155	161	167	173	179	185	192	198	204	210	216	223	229	235	241	247
5'7"	159	166	172	178	185	191	198	204	210	217	223	229	236	242	248	255
5'8"	164	171	177	184	190	197	203	210	217	223	230	236	243	249	256	263
5'9"	169	176	182	189	196	203	209	216	223	230	237	243	250	257	264	270
5'10"	174	181	188	195	202	209	216	223	230	236	243	250	257	264	271	278
5'11"	179	186	193	200	207	215	222	229	236	243	250	258	265	272	279	286
6'0"	184	191	199	206	213	221	228	235	243	250	258	265	272	280	287	294
6'1"	189	197	204	212	219	227	234	242	250	257	265	272	280	287	295	303
6'2"	194	202	210	218	225	233	241	249	256	264	272	280	288	295	303	311
6'3"	200	208	216	224	232	240	247	255	263	271	279	287	295	303	311	319
6'4"	205	213	221	230	238	246	254	262	271	279	287	295	303	312	320	328

11. Sample progress card for a weight control program.

The Progress card measures certain behaviors that help one lose weight. This card is to be carried by a participant at all times. Scores are added up at the end of the day. The card is turned in when you weigh in at the next session and then you are given a new card. Every one should be given an extra card in case they have to miss a session on account of an emergency.

The codes used to score each item are printed on the back of the card. This data is preserved, and if possible, entered into a database computer program for future analysis.

Name:		Week		Start Wt.				End Wt.			
Number	Group	Dates									
Breakfast Score											
Lunch Score											
Between Meal Snack Score											
Foods to Avoid Score											
Walking Score											
Prayer at Meals Score											
Inspirational Reading Score											
Phone Partner Score											
Totals											

Best Weigh Scores

Amount at Each Meal

Skip a meal	81
75% less	7
50% less	6
25% less	4

Walking

hour or more	7
45 minutes	6
30 minutes	5
15 minutes	2

About the same	3		Didn't walk	1
10-25% more	2			
25%+ more	1		**Prayer**	
			3 or more times	4
Between Meal Snacks			2 times	3
No snacks	5		1 time	2
1 snack	3		No prayer	1
2 snacks	2			
3 or more snacks	1		**Inspiration**	
			You found it	3
Foods to Avoid			You did not find it	1
Ate no denied foods	5			
Ate 1 denied food	3		**Phone Your Partner**	
Ate 2 denied foods	?		Yes you called	3
Ate 3 denied foods	1		No you didn't call	1

The top of the card has a place for the participant's name and what group they are in. You may want to assign a number for confidentiality's sake. The dates for the coming week are entered in the top row of small squares. The start weight is the weight at the beginning of each week. At the end of the week the ending weight is entered at weigh-in time and this weight will also be the start weight for the next progress card.

The codes used on the progress card above are arranged in such a way that a higher score at the end of the day is more likely to result in weight loss. At times I have conducted weight control classes where I changed the codes so the better behaviors had lower numbers. When the codes are changed so that lower numbers are desirable for weight loss then the lower the score for the day or the week the more weight you are likely to lose.

Most of the codes are self explanatory. I found that not eating food items a person chose to avoid (except for once a week) was a strong predictor of weight loss. For this reason I now allow people to choose to avoid up to three specific foods during the weight loss program. A participant can have this forbidden food once a week without having to record it as a penalty on the progress card.

On this card I track calling partners, prayer and inspirational reading. I wanted to see if these variables would result in more weight loss than if a person didn't do these behaviors. In other clinics I have only measured eating and exercising variables. Once you design a progress card it is good not to make changes for several sessions as it becomes familiar to those who come back time and again. It is also important for data analysis that the data collected be uniform and comparable from session to session.

These progress cards will get a lot of beating and should be on fairly heavy card stock. I also like to use a hot pink or bright yellow for the cards. It catches a person's eye and reminds them of what they are doing. It also brings up questions from coworkers and family members who see the bright progress card.

Progress cards can be used in exercise programs and stop smoking programs and most any program where behaviors are being changed and can be tracked. A progress card encourages personal accountability and is a daily reminder of what needs to be done. Create you own progress cards. Track different behavioral variables. Assign different values in different ways to each behavior. You will generate data, prove a point and have material to prove the effectiveness of your program.

12. Sample Intake Questionnaire for a weight control program.

This is the type of information that is useful to know in a weight control program.

Name:_____ Today's Date: _____
    (Last)   (First)   (Middle)

Address: _____

Telephone: _____ Date of Birth _____

Circle the number by the answer which is correct:

1.	Sex	1.	Male
		2.	Female

2.	Marital Status	1.	Single
		2.	Married
		3.	Divorced or separated
		4.	Widowed

3.	Highest level of education	1.	Grade school or less.
		2.	Some high school.
		3.	High school graduate.
		4	Some college or trade school.
		5.	College graduate
		6.	Master's degree
		7.	Doctoral degree.

4.	Religious preference	1.	Baptist
		2.	Methodist
		3.	Presbyterian
		4.	Protestant
		5.	Catholic
		6.	Jewish
		7.	Seventh-day Adventist
		8.	Other _____

5. Present weight in indoor   1. Pounds _____
    clothing.

6. Present height without   1. Height _____
    shoes.

7. At what age did you first   1. 0-9   years of age
    become overweight?
                                2. 10-19   years of age

                                3. 20-29   years of age

                                4. 30-39   years of age

                                5. 40+   years of age

8. Has a doctor ever advised   1. Yes
    you to lose weight?
                                2. No

9. What is the most you have   1. _____   Pounds
    ever weighed?

10. What is the most weight   1. 0-9   pounds
    you ever lost by dieting?
                                2. 10-19   pounds

                                3. 20-29   pounds

                                4. 30-39   pounds

                                5. 40-49   pounds

                                6. 50-74   pounds

                                7. 75-100   pounds

                                8. 100+   pounds

11. How many years have you been significantly over-weight?

1. 0-9   years
2. 10-19   years
3. 20-29   years
4. 30-39   years
5. 40+   years.

12. How many pounds would you like to lose at this time?

1. _____   Pounds.

13. Was your father over-weight?

1. Yes
2. No

14. Was your mother over-weight?

1. Yes
2. No

15. Is your spouse overweight?

1. Yes
2. No

16. How often do you eat a good breakfast?

1. Never
2. Occasionally.
3. Frequently
4. Daily. (Most of the time)

17. Which is usually the largest meal of the day?

1. Breakfast
2. Noon meal.
3. Evening meal.

18. How often to you eat
    between meal snacks?

    1. Never

    2. Eat only 1 snack a day between meals.

    3. Eat 2 or 3 snacks a day between meals.

    4. Eat 4 or more snacks a day between meals.

19. Do you drink coffee or tea?

    1. None or rarely.

    2. 1-3 cups or glasses a day.

    3. 4-6 cups or glasses a day.

    4. 7 or more cups or glasses a day.

20. Do you drink soft drinks?
    (Diet or regular)

    1. None or rarely.

    2. 1-2 cans or bottles a day.

    3. 3-4 cans or bottles a day.

    4. 5 or more cans or bottles a day.

21. Do you drink beer, wine or
    other alcoholic drinks?

    1. Never

    2. Rarely (less than once a week)

    3. Occasionally. (once or more a week)

    4. Nearly every day.

22. How much sleep do you
    average each night.

    1. Less than 5 hours.

    2. 5-6 hours

    3. 7-8 hours

    4. 9 or more hours

---

23. Do you have a regular exercise program other than what you get at work.
   1. Yes
   2. No (If no skip to question 26)

24. When you exercise, how much time do you typically spend exercising?
   1. Less than once a week.
   2. 1-2 times a week
   3. 3-4 times a week.
   4. 5 or more times a week.

25. How many minutes do you spend in a typical exercise session?
   1. Less than 15 minutes at a time.
   2. 15-29 minutes at a time
   3. 30-60 minutes at a time.
   4. An hour or more.

26. Before this time about how many times have you made a serious attempt to lose weight by dieting?
   1. None. This is my first real diet.
   2. 1-3 times in the past 5 years.
   3. 4-6 times in the past 5 years.
   4. 7 or more times in the past 5 years.

27. What would you say the probability is that two years from now you will weigh just about the same as you do right now?
   1. Definitely not. I will lose weight now.
   2. Probably not. I hope to lose weight.
   3. Probably yes. I am not sure I can keep it off.
   4. Definitely yes. I can never keep weigh off.

28. Have you been told you have heart trouble?

   1. No (Please explain Yes answers)

   2. Yes. _____

29. Do you get short of breath while walking on the level or climbing one flight of stairs?

   1. No (Please explain Yes answers)

   2. Yes. _____

30. Do you frequently get swelling of the feet or ankles?

   1. No.

   2. Yes _____

31. Do you have high blood pressure?

   1. No.

   2. Yes _____

32. Do you have diabetes?

   1. No

   2. Yes _____

33. Do you have high cholesterol?

   1. No

   2. Yes _____

34. Do you have arthritis in your hips, knees, ankles or feet that limits your walking?

   1. No

   2. Yes _____

35. Do you believe that God helps people lose weight?

   1. No

   2. Yes

   3. Uncertain

You might ask additional questions regarding medications. Is your client taking any prescription or over the counter diet preparations? You might want to ask about blood pressure, heart, cholesterol and other medications.

You might ask questions that determine a person's attitude about losing weight. Questions about a person's understanding about the role of diet, exercise and certain food items might be useful to determine.

13. Sample Last Session and Follow-up Questionnaire for a weight control program.

Name: _____ Date: _____

1. Are you losing weight at the present time?
   1. No.
   2. Yes.

2. Have you lost as much weight as you wanted to?
   1. No
   2. Yes.

3. What is your present weight?
   1. _____ pounds.

4. Have you put on weight since the end of the Weight Management Program?
   1. No
   2. Yes, 5 pounds or less.
   3. Yes, 6-10 pounds.
   4. Yes, 11-20 pounds.
   5. Yes, more than 20 pounds.

5. Compared to your eating habits before the weight management program how are you eating now?

   1. A lot less than before.

   2. Some less than before.

   3. About the same as before.

   4. More than before.

6. Are you eating snacks between meals?

   1. None or rarely. Once a week or less.

   2. Only one snack between meals each day.

   3. Two or three snacks a day.

   4. Four or more snacks a day.

7. Are you eating the food items you were going to avoid?

   1. Never or rarely. Once a week or less.

   2. Less than I used to but regularly.

   3. About the same as usual.

   4. More than ususal.

8. Are you walking, jogging, swimming or bicycle riding?

   1. Never or rarely. Once a week or less.

   2. Two or three times a week.

   3. Four or more times a week.

9. What have you decided to do about your weight in the next 6 months?

   1. Stay about what I weigh now.

   2. Try to lose a few pounds on my own.

   3. Plan to attend the next program at the church.

   4. Plan to try another type of diet program.

10.	Do you make your weight problem a subject of prayer?	1.	Never or rarely. (Once a week or less)
		2.	Occasionally. (2-3 times a week)
		3.	Frequently. (4-6 times a week)
		4.	Daily. (One or more times a day)

14. Small Group Composition Record.

Group Number.   _____

Partners

(Group Leaders)   _____ Phone _____

                     _____ Phone _____

Participants

(Group Members)   _____ Phone _____

                     _____ Phone _____

                     _____ Phone _____

                     _____ Phone _____

                     _____ Phone _____

                     _____ Phone _____

_____ Phone _____

_____ Phone _____

_____ Phone _____

This form is for internal use only. It should be completed at the very first session. Each group leader should have a list of the participants in his or her group. The group members should have the phone numbers of both group leaders so they can be contacted if any of the members has a question or a problem. Group leaders should expect calls from their members, but if the week goes by and some group members have not been heard from, then it is a good thing if the group leader will call those he or she hasn't heard from to see how they are doing and to encourage them to come to the next session.

15. Informed Consent

It is good to have each participant read and sign a consent to attend your program. If you have legal counsel available to you who knows local requirements it would be good to seek a lawyer's advice.

All health programs at the church are educational in nature. You are encouraging people to make changes in their behaviors that promote good health and help them avoid premature sickness and death. All programs are designed to keep the healthy well.

It is not the purpose of any Health Evangelism program to diagnose or treat any specific medical disease. Although health professionals are involved with the program, it is not their purpose to establish any program as a practice of medicine.

Individuals who have significant medical problems who want to take your program should have their physician's permission to attend. A copy of the practitioners recommendation should be kept on file.

Any exercise recommendations you make should be age appropriate and be considered to fall within what a normal person is likely to do in a daily routine. Any diet recommendations made should be considered "balanced" by any general nutritional standards. Medications and therapeutic vitamins and herbs should not be recommended, dispensed or sold at your programs.

Your church should have a general liability insurance policy that covers the activities of church members in the regular conduct of church business. All programs you conduct in the church should have the voted and recorded authorization of the church board making your program an official function of the local church. Health practitioners who help should be covered by their own liability insurance.

Our society is litigious. God wants us to reach out and help whoever we can. We should do so wisely. God will bless and God will protect.

Men's Health

0-595-31243-8

1. October

Slots
— growing
Diet

Oct Ag.

Printed in the United States
133733LV00006B/34-60/A